Praise for *Animal Healing*

"[*Animal Healing* features] a detailed guide to gaining greater connection with our animals using healing techniques, including reiki, crystals, and Bach flower remedies. [You'll discover] fascinating case studies too, most of which tug at the heart strings. Unputdownable."
—Liza Goddard, actress

"This beautiful book gently and eloquently unwraps the mysteries of animal communication and healing and guides the reader to compassionate understanding. Niki's extraordinary personal story, and the accounts of animals she has helped, affirm the effectiveness of her methods and teachings.... *Animal Healing* is inspirational, uplifting, educational, and ultimately is, in itself, a healing facilitator."
—Lisa Tenzin-Dolma, author and principal of The International School for Canine Psychology & Behaviour, Ltd

"This book is enthralling and you'll be unable to put it down... This book will open up a door to your soul; I urge you to open that door and begin your own special journey into not only helping animals, but in finding your true self."
—Leigh Taylor-Shayle, equine dentist WWE (Idaho) and founder of Straight From the Horse's Mouth

"A truly amazing book. Following Niki's journey to how she became an animal healer was a very inspirational and enjoyable read; Niki's essence really radiates throughout this book. It offers a great understanding of the role healing and holistic therapies have to play in the animal kingdom. This book takes you step by step though many holistic practices and teaches how to apply these yourself... [It's] not only a great read but a fantastic reference manual."
—Vickie China, mCAAM, canine myotherapist and laser specialist

"Thought provoking and inspiring us all to connect on a deeper level."
—Barbara Wilkinson, trustee of the Herb Society

"For anyone who shares their life with an animal companion, [*Animal Healing*] will make invaluable and inspiring reading... This is a must-have, step-by-step book for anyone, professional or layman, wanting to keep their pets healthy in mind, body and spirit in a holistic way."
—Molly Farrar, founder of Feline Care Cat Rescue

"Each method [Niki J. Senior] uses is explained with case studies and new techniques are described in clear and easy-to-read detail. This wonderful book allows you to heal and relax while gaining a deeper connection and understanding of your pet... I will be using Niki's advice and techniques for many years to come."
—Anna Georghallides, owner and editor of *Paws Up* magazine

"[*Animal Healing* includes] a combination of anecdotes, success stories, personal battles, science, therapies, how-to instruction, and self-care... by the time you have finished, your love for your animal, yourself, and for all of life will have reached new vibrations, new connections, and higher energies—you will already be healing your animal before you know it! Now, that's magic."
—Isla Fishburn, PhD, MBiolSci, BSc, founder of Kachina Canine

"As a professional vet, I found this book an enlightening approach to holistic animal health and understand how complementary and veterinary methods can work in synergy."
—Bernd Wittorf, MRCVS, veterinarian, Freie Universität Berlin

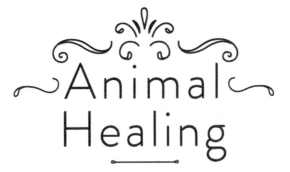

About the Author

Niki J. Senior (Norfolk, United Kingdom) has taught professional animal healing courses and animal therapy training since 1997. She was awarded training school status in 2010 for her animal therapy training courses, which are some of the only diploma-level classes of this kind available in the UK. She also created AniScentia, her canine nutrition and herbal remedy company, and Animal Essentia, a complete professional practitioner training course using tree essences. Visit her online at www.AnimalMagicTraining.com.

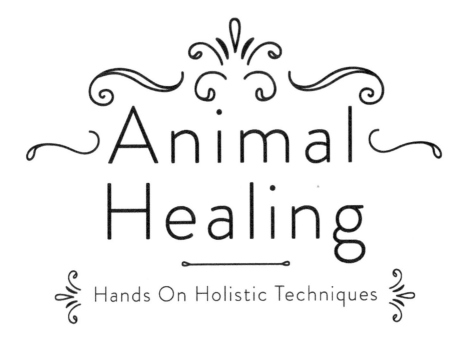

Animal Healing

Hands On Holistic Techniques

Niki J. Senior

Llewellyn Worldwide
Woodbury, Minnesota

FIRST EDITION
Second Printing, 2022

Book design by Bob Gaul
Cover design by Shira Atakpu

Llewellyn Publications is a registered trademark of Llewellyn Worldwide Ltd.

Library of Congress Cataloging-in-Publication Data

Names: Senior, Niki J., author.
Title: Animal healing : hands-on holistic techniques / Niki J. Senior.
Description: First Edition. | Woodbury : Llewellyn Worldwide, Ltd., 2018.
Identifiers: LCCN 2018033815 (print) | LCCN 2018037585 (ebook) | ISBN
   9780738758473 (ebook) | ISBN 9780738757773 (alk. paper)
Subjects: LCSH: Holistic veterinary medicine. | Energy medicine. | Precious
   stones—Therapeutic use. | Human-animal relationships.
Classification: LCC SF745.5 (ebook) | LCC SF745.5 .S46 2018 (print) | DDC
   636.089/55—dc23
LC record available at https://lccn.loc.gov/2018033815

Llewellyn Publications
A Division of Llewellyn Worldwide Ltd.
2143 Wooddale Drive
Woodbury, MN 55125-2989
www.llewellyn.com

Printed in the United States of America

This book is dedicated to all the animals past and present that have shared my physical space and the inner place of my heart. You entwined my heart and soul and showed me immeasurable understanding and unrivaled friendship, and have taught me all that is worth knowing with purity and compassion. I am humbled by your love, and without your guidance, your intelligence, and your wisdom, none of this would have been possible.

For Saskia: my whole world.

Contents

Acknowledgments

I would like to express my gratitude to the many people who saw me make my (often arduous) way through the writing of this book. Thank you to all involved, but especially to Louis, my heart and soul. Who would have known that when I left everything behind on the 26th of February, 2000, to move in together after spending just ten hours in your company, that we'd be here in Norfolk living our rural dream? Thank you for your love, your encouragement, your unfettered support, your friendship, and all your delicious culinary creations made to sustain me through the writing of this book. "Swallows and Amazons—Forever"! My soul mate—I love you deeply.

To Helen Fletcher, who trawled through this book for many hours, correcting and editing. Helen—my friend, my editor, and one of the most genuine people I have ever met. To Mia Fletcher, the daughter I never had; thank you for being the special you. To Tom Fletcher; thank you for the loan of your guinea pigs for student training practical sessions.

To Liza Goddard, the actress and conservationist; thank you for writing the foreword to this book, for being a wonderful friend, and for attending and promoting my courses. I am honored by our mutual love of earth-based medicine. I also offer thanks to your lovely daughter Sophie, for introducing us.

To Lesley Pasuto, for supporting and encouraging me in everything I do; you are so much more than a friend.

Many thanks go to my hundreds of students, now graduates worldwide, for allowing me to share my passion and walk alongside you on this magical journey. To my students of the future, I look forward to forging new friendships.

To Valerie Crofts and the gorgeous gentle soul that was Poppy, the Rottweiler. She taught my students how to heal, showed them the way, and will be forever my guide.

Much gratitude goes out to all who have endorsed this book.

For Saskia, my Tibetan prayer dog; through you I know the immeasurable depth of love. Saskia: my heart, my soul, my life.

To all the animals that have crossed my path in search of healing, you have indeed healed my heart and soul.

I beg forgiveness of all those whose names I have failed to mention.

I give thanks to life itself; I'm enjoying this journey. Thanks for giving me a second chance!

A Life in Animals

Reflections by Liza Goddard, Actress and Conservationist

Ireland has some breathtaking scenery and is a lovely place to spend a holiday; however, I wonder how many people return home to the UK with a Connemara pony in tow? I did. The fact is, I've gathered many wonderful animal companions over the years from my travels, and often I didn't have to journey that far.

My earliest memory was with a pony called Cassie. I was aged about eighteen months and remember sitting upon Cassie, smiling; this was the start of my love for horses. My other friend at this time was a beautiful Boxer dog called Bella. We too shared many magical moments together; one such moment was sat at the side of her with a trowel in my hand and the both of us digging in the flower beds.

When I was a little older we moved house. The house was in the middle of a wood and we were lucky enough to have a menagerie of animals, including a Poodle and a pet goose named Sidney. Sidney was a quite a character, as he insisted on accompanying me to the bus stop, then taking a detour via a few neighbors for treats on his return journey home. Visitors to our house often took their lives in their hands when

Sidney was about, as he'd peck at their car tires, daring them to set foot out of the car. They often had to beep their horns to alert us to move Sidney out of their way.

When Sidney was about, nobody dared mention the word "picnic." We'd sneak out of the house and set the food down on our picnic rug. Then halfway through eating we'd see Sidney's head appear from the corner of the house, and he'd stampede his way towards us and ransack the sandwiches and scones.

A few years later, along came another pony, Mousey, a former whipper-in pony who was the ultimate guardian. With her I felt totally safe. I enjoyed living in my imaginary world and Mousey enjoyed our adventures. We'd ride out together, and I'd pretend to be a roundhead or even Joan of Arc with my wooden sword in hand. Mousey even supported my idea to be a stunt woman, as I'd practice falling off her whilst still holding the reins. I never broke a single bone; she was so gentle with me. Because of this, friends would ask to ride her, but Mousey only wanted me to be on her back. Friends would take her out for a ride and after half an hour or so, back she came, without her rider. It transpired that she'd thrown them halfway through the outing! Along with the dislike of being ridden by anyone but me, Mousey loathed gymkhanas. The only race she enjoyed participating in was "the vegetarian race": a very odd race which involved galloping down to the end of the field, the horse munching an apple and rider eating digestive biscuits. We won every time.

I have been an actress since the 1960s and I'm sure people of a certain age in Australia remember the television program *Skippy*. I played the teenager Clarissa "Clancy" Merrick and appeared in nearly fifty episodes. Everyone loved Skippy the bush kangaroo, but in reality there were around twenty Skippys. It was a fun period of my life, and the first time I had worked with animals professionally. The breed of kangaroo we used for the program was the Eastern Grey Kangaroo, as they have excellent temperaments. Unlike the programs featuring animals today, we didn't have trainers back then, and I remember the kangaroos toileting everywhere; in forty degree heat, the smell wasn't a pleasant one! They were very fond of running away at every opportunity, and on many occasions we'd be filming and just out of camera shot there would be an animal handler holding on to the tail of the "Skippy" we were using for the scene, just to make sure he'd stay put for the duration; it wouldn't be allowed now! At the end of the filming week there would be a prize for the guy who caught the most Skippys and returned them back to base.

When the kangaroos weren't working in television scenes, they enjoyed lying in sacks because it mimicked their mothers' pouch. The animals that weren't so cooperative during filming were wombats and emus. We discovered they were all quite savage! The koala was different again, so laid back and obliging; in fact, we did a whole scene with a koala sitting on an ironing board!

Prior to my move to Australia and my work on *Skippy*, I'd attended the Arts Education Trust in the UK. As it was a long commute from Farnham, where I lived with my family, to London, I stayed with my parents' friends Brenda Ulrich (a portrait artist) and her husband, David. Their lifestyle sparked my whole interest in the holistic world. These friends were advocates of Adele Davis's work and her philosophy for vitamin supplementation and vital nutrition through healthy food; I became converted to a new way of healthy living.

I then discovered yoga, and this led me on to look at many different forms of spirituality in the years that followed. After reading a series of books I discovered shamanism. I enrolled on an introductory course and was hooked. For the past twelve years I've practiced shamanism, and this has deepened my connective spirituality greatly.

Connecting both mind and body is vastly important to me, and in recent years in the UK I have enjoyed working alongside a naturopath and cranial chiropractor. After each session I feel totally balanced, like all my energy is flowing in the direction it should.

Becoming aware of my own requirements in holistic health allowed me to evaluate the needs of my own animals, especially my rescue dogs Donald and Honey, who had suffered greatly before coming to me. Each, sadly, has now passed on, and I live with Holly, a Spangledor, and Violet, a Yorkshire Terrier, both rescues as well.

Through my daughter, Sophie, I met Niki. After reading about her vast knowledge in the subject of animal wellness, I leapt at the chance to attend one of her courses in animal healing; I knew this could benefit my own animals greatly. I was fully engaged from the start, as her courses are well laid-out, easy to follow, interesting, and fun too. Consequently, I enrolled on two further courses with Niki and I am now also a practitioner of Reiki.

Hands-on healing helped not only my rescue dog Honey, but also Donald, who was an adorable black Labrador. When I met Donald I thought he was a greyhound cross because he was seriously malnourished. He had been living with a foster carer who also had a Staffordshire Bull Terrier, whose tendency was to act aggressively towards Donald. Consequently, when Donald came to me, he was a dog experiencing many anxieties. Because of prolonged stress, his stomach had developed an inability to keep in nutrients and he suffered from constant diarrhea.

In spring 2015 he started a very strange thing: eating wood. After a little research I decided to offer him some mineral supplements, and he magically stopped this. With love, care, and commitment, Donald made a complete recovery and was a typical loving Labrador. However, unlike most Labradors, he didn't much care for water; he preferred to watch cricket! My husband, David, only needed to say "cricket" and off he ran to settle himself down in front of the match.

From experience, I believe many domesticated animals (dogs in particular) have a very stressful lifestyle. Most dogs live in completely unnatural environments, spending far too much time indoors or on their own. When I was a child, dogs were let out in the morning and would meet up with their "gang" members, run around, and then be home again for tea. Nowadays dogs are indoors whilst their owners are working, get offered only a short walk when they arrive home, and then are once again shut in the kitchen at bedtime. Obviously, this will lead to behavior that is not conducive to their mental, emotional, and physical wellbeing.

At one stage in my life I had nine rescue dogs in total. Canine companions have brought me so much pleasure over the years. Through my love of all animals, I became patron of the Hawk and Owl Trust, a UK charity dedicated to conserving owls and birds of prey in the wild. I am also patron Dogs Trust.

I have thoroughly enjoyed reading Niki's book and have learnt so much from her infectious enthusiasm. When Niki asked me to write the foreword to her book, I felt honored and excited to be asked. Her training, along with this book, has inspired me to progress with my healing journey and to further enrich my relationships with my own animals—including Tufty, the rescue pony from Connemara, who is now aged twenty-seven. It is my turn to give something back to all my rescued animals, and with the help of this book, I believe I can achieve it.

Introduction

By the standards set by modern medicine, holistic healing shouldn't work. However, we know that it does. We don't quite understand how or why, but when we witness the miraculous results of simply the laying-on of hands, of herbal remedies, or of placing a crystal near our pet, we become converted to trusting in the old ways of medical treatment.

Our ancestors didn't have access to the medicine we have today; they relied upon natural sources to provide their healing, be it plants or trees, earth or clay, voice or hands. Modern medicine has progressed greatly into the science we know today, and great leaps have been made in veterinary medicine, which has ended much suffering and saved the lives of our beloved animal companions. Consequently, the old ways were pushed aside in favor of new conventional treatment. However, pet owners have begun to realize that orthodox medicine alone often only treats the symptoms and not the root cause of illness, something which holistic medicine works to provide.

Generally, people who use conventional medicine usually do not seek treatment until their animal becomes ill. Within conventional medicine there is little emphasis on preventive treatment. Drugs, surgery, and radiation therapy are among the key tools for dealing with the symptoms of illness and certainly do not address the cause.

In contrast, holistic animal medicine focuses on preventing illness and maintaining the health and well-being of an animal. It views good health as a balance of all body systems: mental, emotional, and spiritual as well as physical. In complementary medicine, all aspects of an animal are seen as interrelated: a principle called "holism," meaning a "state of wholeness." Disharmony in the above aspects of being is thought to stress the body and perhaps lead to sickness.

Natural animal medicine following a holistic approach views illness and disease as an imbalance of the mind and body that is expressed on the physical, emotional, and mental levels of an animal. Although allopathy does recognize that many physical symptoms have mental components (for example, emotional stress might promote an animal to demonstrate negative behavioral changes), its approach is generally to suppress the symptoms on both the physical and psychological levels. Natural medicine assesses the symptoms as a sign or reflection of a deeper instability within the animal, and subsequently tries to restore the physical and mental harmony which will then alleviate the initial symptoms.

Holistic medicine recognizes that the human and animal body is superbly equipped to resist disease and heal injuries. But when disease does take hold, or an injury occurs, the first instinct in holistic healing is to see what might be done to strengthen those natural resistance and healing agents so they can act against the disease more effectively. Results are not expected to occur overnight. But neither are they expected to occur at the cost of dangerous side effects, which is often the case with orthodox treatment.

Holistic healing treats the underlying cause of illness through a variety of natural healing methods, which are applied with empathy and compassion and are often noninvasive. Its focus is to look at all aspects of the animal and to be open to using a variety of treatments if necessary, along with conventional veterinary medicine. During a holistic treatment, communication between the animal, its owner, and the therapist is emphasized.

I have practiced as a professional animal therapist since 1996 and have worked alongside many vets, teaching them how holistic energy medicine can be implemented into modern medical practice. I also receive many client referrals from veterinary practices. I recognize that the most modern veterinary techniques, such as ultrasound, sophisticated laboratory tests, and surgical procedures, are necessary in caring for animals. Even though I wholeheartedly trust holistic medicine, one hundred percent, my veterinarian is always the first point of contact when my own animals are sick. Without their experience in diagnosis techniques, I would be unable to treat my animals effectively and efficiently. Complementary medical practitioners such as myself do not diagnose illness.

More vets are implementing holistic methods of healing, and many of the graduates of my animal therapy courses are continuously finding themselves being offered practice rooms within veterinary surgeries across the UK. Animal medical professionals, pet owners, and the animals themselves are experiencing holistic energy medicine working, often where conventional medicine has not. Chronic debilitating illnesses, common ailments, aches, pains, and everything in between have responded to energy medicine practices. Energy medicine is shedding light on the true nature of health and disease and offering solutions to seemingly intractable animal health problems, often leaving owners more attuned to their animal than they thought possible.

Discovering Wholeness—My Aim for This Book

Through writing this book, I aim to teach you the true essence of animal medicine and its contribution to the interspecies bond. You will discover the complete animal chakra system, including the all-knowing "butterfly chakra," and learn how to use a pendulum during hands-on healing to detect chakra energetic imbalances and emotional trauma.

You will discover how Reiki can help maintain your animal's health and vitality. The wisdom of the crystal kingdom in healing physical illness and injury, and in aiding emotional healing, will also be discussed, and you'll be introduced to the way essences from flowers and trees can be used to heal. We'll delve into how animals communicate with us, and turn the key to understanding the needs and wishes of animals through a variety of "Step by Step" exercises. If you're interested in becoming a professional animal healer and furthering your knowledge of the many ways we can alleviate animal illness, this book will give you a deeper insight.

From dogs and cats to horses, birds, and even wildlife, my goal is to help you understand and utilize the power of a hands-on, holistic approach—to heal, to bring positivity, and to deepen your bond with the animals in your life. If you have a passion for animals and you wish to make a considerable and appreciable difference to their lives, and in so doing enhance your connection to your own soul center, let nothing hold you back. Congratulations on buying this book; this is your first step to wholeness.

When I said to my mum at the age of seven that I was put on the planet to help care for the animals, little did I know that over forty years on I would be doing just that; not only as a healer and therapist, but also as a teacher, helping others learn how to heal compassionately and communicate with purity. My cat Timmy taught me to understand, to listen, and to heal. He was instrumental in my whole journey in the realm of healing.

It is my desire for this book to help you, the reader, rediscover a part of yourself that has remained hidden or undiscovered until now. It is also my desire to assist everyone who shares a true passion for animal wellness to harness the universal energy that links us all together.

1
Unexpected Connections

There's a feral cat with the most enticing, rich, emerald-green eyes beside me as I write these words. Or rather, he *was* feral …

It was November 2014, and my partner, Louis, asked me to take a look in our barn. As I peered out through the conservatory window, a black-and-white "tuxedo" cat looked back at me. His face was as black as the night, and he had the most striking long, snow-white whiskers. "Muddle looks different," Louis remarked.

Now, Muddle is another story; he was a stray cat who was left behind when neighbors moved out of the county. Refusing to live at a nearby farm in spite of their efforts to entice him with food, he adopted us and we had no say in the matter; that was over six years ago. Declining to set foot inside our cottage despite much persuasion, Muddle is nicely set up inside the barn with a heated bed, a thick single duvet, and numerous cozy fleeces—oh, and of course three good meals a day.

How on earth my husband couldn't tell that the new visitor wasn't Muddle I will never know, especially as the newbie had a large portion of his left ear missing. Most charities, when neutering and spaying feral cats, use the ear snip method to indicate a feral that has been treated, to save the cats the trauma of being trapped a second time. This procedure is called trap, neuter, return—TNR for short. At this point we didn't know if this feline visitor was male or female, though I did have a strong inclination he might be male.

I opened the conservatory door to place some food out by the barn entrance where this stranger was sitting, but he obviously found our hospitality too overwhelming and fled up the magnolia tree and over the fence. I hoped he'd return. The next day, around about the same time, he appeared again, and then the next day too; in fact, he returned every dinner time for the next few months.

As the weeks passed by, the cat became braver and would sit and wait under the silver birch tree by the barn, peering between the bare branches, waiting for me to go indoors after putting out food before he'd venture out of hiding for his meal. I asked around our village if he belonged to anyone and fly-posted and leaflet-dropped, but nobody came forward to claim him.

I purchased a second heated pad and equipped an old cat carrier with fleeces over the winter months; I hated to think of him having nowhere warm and cozy to sleep during the long winter nights. I prayed that he and Muddle wouldn't fight; my prayers were answered because they never did.

Spring came around, and in the third week of March I was overjoyed when Tippy (as we'd named him due to the ear tip snip) allowed me to make physical contact. I hovered my fingers over his back and touched his tail as he swept past me en route to his feed bowl. I was so emotional that I sat on the cold floor of the barn and cried. After five months he'd actually trusted me enough to let me touch him, albeit for a fleeting moment.

As I sat upon the floor observing him eat, I saw that his posture didn't look quite right; he seemed to be shifting his weight from pad to pad. Looking closely at his legs, then at his paws, I saw a protruding growth attached to his left hind-leg pad; it looked really swollen and was bulging open. My tears of joy soon turned to sadness as I wondered how long he'd been suffering with this, if he was in pain, and how on earth I was going to treat it; until Tippy, I'd had no experience of truly feral cats.

I didn't sleep at all that night and I feared the worst. After speaking with a good friend who is a veterinary receptionist, along with showing her blurry photographs of Tippy's foot via email (blurry due to my inability to get close to Tippy with my camera), she confirmed my suspicions that it could be a tumor.

I had no other option than to trap him, which meant throwing a towel over him and launching him into our old dog crate. The night had come and this wild-natured cat was now fighting, spitting, hissing, and wailing, trying to free himself from the confinement of the metal trap. We put a blanket over the pen to help calm him down, and I sobbed. All the trust I had built up over the past five months had come crashing down. I'd betrayed Tippy, and for this I felt terribly guilty.

The next day the vet assured me I had done the right thing in capturing him, because as she looked closely at the growth, she warned me that there was a distinct possibility that it was cancer and Tippy might even need a leg amputation; all was dependent on the results of the histology report. She advised that at the very least he would lose a toe; however, should the tumor have spread inwards to other tissue or bone, amputation would be the only option to save the life of this cat. I prepared myself for bad news and tried not to become too attached to Tippy; after all, he was feral and we might never have a normal feline/human relationship anyway.

When I collected him later that day, the veterinarian advised that she had removed the cancerous growth, sent it for a histology report, and actually managed to save his toe! I was thrilled, yet extremely worried at the same time; I had here a feral cat, unable to walk and needing to be confined to our spare room for a good few weeks to recover.

An apprehensive two weeks passed until Tippy was free of stitches. The vet had made three home visits, and his wound had healed nicely and without infection. He also had a good appetite and was using a litter tray. Furthermore, his histology results couldn't have been more positive; the tumor was an external growth so no leg amputation was needed!

During his recuperation I applied distant healing with Tippy, due to his inability to trust hands-on touch. I wanted healing to be as non-invasive as possible. I sat a few feet away from his cage and directed healing energy to various parts of his body. He was extremely responsive and I knew from observing his movements that he found the energy comforting. He pressed parts of his body that were in need of healing to the cage bars. In addition, I placed some basic crystal therapy grids and relevant gemstones at strategic points around his room to enhance positive energy and stimulate his physical and mental vitality. I often caught him looking up to the top of the curtain pole or underneath my desk, the very places I'd placed the crystals.

Hannah the vet was amazed at Tippy's progress and gave him the all clear after six weeks. The holistic healing approach had enabled this cat to progress with trust, and it had accelerated his healing on every level, and with amazing results too. Unbelievably, less than two months previously, Tippy had been a feral, filled with fear and mistrust and struggling to walk, scrounging for meals. Now he'd turned into a beautiful cat, a happy and well-rounded indoor snuggle-puss.

We are unsure of his age, but Tippy has captured not just my heart, but that of our dog too; they're the best of friends. Tippy purrs, plays, and insists I rub his tummy; it's like he's always been here. In fact, I feel as though I've met Tippy before; in a previous life? Who knows?

My Formative Years

I was born in the year of decimalization, into a hard-working Yorkshire family. It was early January when my mum went into labor, and the whole region was experiencing a severe snowstorm, which resulted in a power cut at the hospital. On that cold night, just days after Christmas, I came into the world at 8:00 p.m. I guess from the moment I was born on that dark winter's night, I journeyed on to seek only light in my life.

I was taken home by my parents to a house that looked much like those on the rest of the street: a cream-colored, textured affair with a shared driveway. My father was a builder and my mother an assistant in a news agency.

As an only child, throughout my younger years I suffered from anxiety and severe bouts of fear. My parents back then had a turbulent and somewhat unsettled relationship, which led me to spend much of my early years worrying about the people who were supposed to keep me safe. I felt I had nobody to confide in.

In the early hours of an autumnal morning, aged about five, I remember being wrenched from my warm and comforting bed by my mother and taken out to walk the cold, blustery streets; my parents had had yet another heated argument. This was a regular occurrence and understandably it left me feeling rather unnerved. I quickly became an introverted child and I lacked confidence in many social situations. I was bullied at school for not participating in group activities, yet I just didn't feel part of any group; I much preferred to be on my own. I lacked the emotional support of siblings, and my parents were often too busy for me to express my concerns to. I understand this to be the very start of my deep connection with the animal kingdom. I found it hard to relate to most people, much preferring to be in the company of animals. I felt they listened to me, understood me, supported me, and asked for nothing in return.

Spiritual Companion

Just before my ninth birthday I discovered a friend who'd keep a watchful eye over me. He offered me security and comfort in his nightly visitations. His name was Dr. Watson. This chap was a tall, elderly gentleman who wore a striking claret-colored cravat, a tailcoat, and a taller-than-tall black top hat. With his silver-topped walking cane in his right hand, he appeared before me every night, always as dusk fell. Dr. Watson would appear at the foot of my bed, looking over at me tucked up beneath my eiderdown. I found comfort in those nightly appearances, and after we spoke (telepathically) he would touch his nose twice and disappear through my bedroom wall. I confided my worries and concerns to Dr. Watson and knew he understood me. My parents must have thought I was a strange little girl, no doubt putting my experiences down to an overactive imagination, but I know what I saw, and to me Dr. Watson *was* real.

Playing the Piper

A few years earlier, when I was aged four, my parents named me "the Tiny Pied Piper." Nursery school was around two miles away, so Mum and I would set off walking there. Mum would find herself shooing away cats and dogs that were tagging along behind us (in the early seventies, many dogs were allowed to roam freely around the streets). Cats would jump down from fence posts, dogs would run out from bushes and undergrowth, all wanting to make friends with me, as I did with them. Whilst Mum was waving her arms around trying to dissuade them from following us, I'd communicate with the animals. I didn't really understand what I was doing at the time and thought everyone could speak to animals, mind to mind. I'd send out thoughts of safety, asking them to go back home and not to follow us for fear of them being knocked over and killed by speeding traffic. I knew they understood me and off they went.

Jason

Before the summer holidays, when I was seven years old, I made another unexpected connection with animals. Mum was late in collecting me from junior school. All the other children had gone home and I was becoming anxious as I waited alone outside the school gates. However, my thoughts soon eased when a very handsome Dalmatian dog came to sit beside me. I stroked his head and he made quiet snuffling noises. It was as though this dog knew my fears and was trying to help alleviate my anxiety. He was offering me security and wanted to keep me safe until Mum arrived. I later discovered that the dog's name was Jason, and that he lived a few houses away from my nan and granddad, just five minutes' walk from school.

From the day Jason first introduced himself at the school gates, we became the best of friends. Nan had a beautiful ornamental rosebush in her garden, arched over the front gate. It towered over me and the scent was truly delicious. It was like nothing I had ever smelled, or have even smelled since. Whenever I use pure essential oil of rose, it conjures up some wonderful childhood memories of my nan's garden, and the fun I shared there with Jason.

I would arrive at Nan's house, a 1930s semi-detached with a long rear garden and vegetable plot beyond, and Jason would leap over the garden gate to join me on my picnic blanket upon the grass. One particular summer's day, I snapped off a number of fragrant rose heads and joined them together with bits of colored ribbon and sticky tape to make a headdress. I placed it on Jason's head and said the crown made him the king of all dogs; I swear I saw him smile. Because Jason enjoyed dressing up, I spied and took an old waistcoat that belonged to granddad hanging over the washing line. Granddad wasn't pleased to have spent two hours looking for his "best" waistcoat only to find Jason wearing it!

When I wasn't with Jason at Nan's, I was home with friends, but all my friends on our street liked to take the neighbors' toddlers for walks in their pushchairs. I just wasn't interested in doing this. I'd look out of the lounge window to see my friend Mandy wheeling around a toddler in a blue-and-white striped buggy. One day I said to Mum, "I'm never going to have babies; I'm going to look after animals." Mum conveyed a stern look and expressed that at the age of seven I couldn't make such an important life decision and that I would change my mind as I grew older, but I never did.

My thoughts as a child were only for animals; I was interested in very little else. In those days we didn't have computers, DVDs, or gaming consoles, so when I received a portable black-and-white television for my tenth birthday I was thrilled. I locked myself in my bedroom with my skinny black cat, Timmy—whom you will meet in the next chapter—and watched nothing but animal documentaries, *Blue Peter* (for the animals that appeared on the show), and *Animal Magic*, which was my favorite! Johnny Morris quickly became my hero; I thought that the animals were really speaking to him, just as I could hear the animals speaking with me. I also wrote to the TV program *Jim'll Fix It* and asked if they could fix it for me to spend a day at a zoo with the big cats and stroke a lion or tiger, but I never received a reply, thankfully.

Scottie

Any people who happened to pass by our house were quickly stopped in their tracks if walking their dog; I *needed* to stroke it! My parents had constantly refused to buy me a canine companion, so I decided that if I couldn't have a dog of my own, then I would jolly well pack my bags and run away to a house that did. I ran away but I didn't stray far, going to my friend's grandparents' house just two streets away. They had a small West Highland Terrier named Scottie who frantically licked my face whenever he saw me. I was content for the whole afternoon—playing games with Scottie, giving him his dinner, grooming him, and sharing great conversation—until I thought about my cat, Timmy, back home. I began to miss Timmy terribly. After a final cuddle from Scottie I was homeward bound, but on the corner of our street I saw my angry-faced mum appear. Apparently my parents had been combing the streets looking for me. Timmy head-rubbed me upon my return, making welcoming trilling noises. I vowed never to run away and leave him again.

The Goldfish

Mum and Dad thought I was more than a little odd with my animal obsession, and looking back I guess I didn't appear to be like other children. Granddad knew this too. He'd often say I'd been on planet earth before and that I was an old soul. I didn't understand what he meant back then; I just knew, even as a young child, that I was put on earth to give something back to the animal kingdom for all it gave to me.

I was looking through my bedroom window one day when I heard a distant voice, followed by the sound of horses' hooves upon the tarmac. A large shire horse came into view, pulling a cart laden with material and old clothing. I caught sight of something hanging from the cart, swinging in the breeze. As I couldn't quite make it out, I closed my window and went outside to take a closer look. Oh my! Individual plastic bags tied with pieces of wire, containing a goldfish in each one. The thought of them being jolted around by the motion of the cart made me feel sick. The man driving the cart was called Danny. Danny White was a rag-and-bone man who collected folks' old and tatty clothing, for what purpose was unknown, and in return would offer a goldfish to any child who ran out and gave him their old clothes.

As I stood stroking the great big horse, I became aware that not all of these goldfish were going to go to loving homes. I wanted to take them all home; I wanted to rescue them. My mum handed over a pair of Dad's old overalls and I was presented with one of the goldfish. I couldn't wait to get him indoors and release him from the confinement of the plastic bag. Mum didn't have a goldfish bowl so we put him in a large fruit bowl; he darted around and to me he looked a little stressed. Even at this young age I thought how wrong it was to offer a living creature in return for some tatty, stained rags.

Without hesitation I ran outside just as Danny was leaving. "Wait," I called out, and he pulled the horse and cart to a halt. "Why do you give away goldfish?" I asked. "Cos they don't cost me owt," he replied. I explained how wrong it was and how these fish might not end up in caring environments. He looked quite puzzled, and with a condescending chuckle he took out his whip, tapped it on the bottom of the horse, tightened the reigns, and trotted away. I felt very upset that my words had fallen on deaf ears and came back indoors, putting Timmy upon my lap for comfort. He purred and nuzzled under my chin as I wondered what other action I could take.

I loved poetry when I was young, and still do (especially the works of W. B. Yeats and Byron), though seldom do I now have the chance to pen my own words like I did as a child. After the goldfish episode, I took out my exercise book, home to all my poetry and personal notes, and wrote some simple but heartfelt words about the plight of my newly liberated goldfish. I may have been only eight or nine, but even then I was aware how all creatures can suffer at the hands of human beings.

Months later, I was playing a game of rounders with the boys on our street when trotting up the road came Danny and his horse again. I shuddered and didn't want to look at the cart as it drew closer, for fear of seeing those goldfish again. However, festooned on the back of the cart was a glorious display of brightly colored balloons. I looked inside the cart for the goldfish and I couldn't see any. I asked Danny why there were no fish. "I thought about what you said, young miss, so I decided to offer balloons instead; plus it makes my cart more attractive." I smiled and felt a sense of joy in my heart. Danny *had* actually listened to my plea and had taken action.

Speaking Up

Many years passed and I became a teenager. I developed an interest in music and in one band in particular—the Smiths. I would listen to their music at every opportunity; in fact, the Smiths helped me find peace through the turbulent years of adolescence. The title track from their latest album at the time, *Meat Is Murder*, struck a chord with me.

Overnight, I became vegetarian. My parents thought it was just a fad and that I'd go back to eating meat, but I knew differently. Mum tried to get me to eat her homemade beef burgers, but the stench of them cooking made me physically sick. I found it hard to believe that people failed to make the connection between a pork chop and a pig, or see that the steak on their plate was once a cow that had suffered an agonizing death to make it to their fork. After many months of reasoning, I just couldn't work out the answer. I tried to see if there were allowances to be made for the deaths of animals in terms of the food chain, like overpopulation or planetary benefits, but there were none that I could deduce for the mass slaughter of millions of innocent creatures killed in the name of food.

Over two and a half million cattle, ten million pigs, fourteen and a half million sheep and lambs, eighty million fish, and nine hundred million birds are slaughtered each year for food in the UK alone.[1] Most animals in Britain are stunned before being slaughtered, which involves sending a large voltage through the animal's brain. How on earth could any sane human being with any sort of compassion for animal welfare think that this torture is acceptable?

Even as I write this book I have a lump in my throat. I am not suggesting that anyone reading these pages must turn to vegetarianism; all I ask is that you think about what you are actually eating, and to spare a thought for how the animal experienced great suffering to make it onto your plate. Paul McCartney once said, "If slaughterhouses had

---

1   Humane Slaughter Association. https://www.hsa.org.uk/faqs/general.

glass walls, everyone would be a vegetarian."[2] I totally agree. Having a deep connection to animals since childhood helped me develop my awareness of their suffering and pain, and as the years passed I knew I needed to do even more to help them.

The Animal's Voice

All animals deserve to have their basic needs met; love, food, and security are just three of these needs. They ask for little else. Animals have no voice, so it's up to us human beings to listen to them in a variety of other ways, mainly through our conscience. Along with turning to vegetarianism, I became an avid campaigner for numerous organizations that supported many facets of animal welfare. Initially I supported the work of an organization that put an end to the breeding of guinea pigs that were supplied to the pharmaceutical research industry. My part in the campaign was to distribute flyers by post to other animal welfare campaigners, as there was no internet in those days. I raised awareness about what was actually happening within the world of animal vivisection, and so many people were shocked to discover that scientific experimentation wasn't just limited to rats. The guinea pigs in my particular campaign were living in dirty, barren, and crowded conditions, covered in their own excrement inside huge breeding sheds, as well as trying to survive amongst other dead and dying guinea pigs. Due to the many people working to raise awareness, this particular establishment was thankfully eventually closed down.

I recall another joyous moment, not long after this successful campaign, when I was nineteen and had just bought my first house. I picked up a call from a woman who was the leader of a campaign to close down a cat-breeding establishment in Oxfordshire. Yet again, these cats were bred to be tortured in the name of scientific research. Our lengthy campaign finally came to an end with the news that we had all been waiting

---

2   Narration for "Glass Walls" video, PETA, 2012.

for: the RSPCA had been sent in to rescue and try to rehome some eight hundred cats. The campaign resulted in another satisfying conclusion.

Most people aren't aware that domestic animals such as cats and dogs are used for experimentation too. There are more animals than rats, rabbits, and mice that are needlessly destroyed and tortured every year, all in the name of scientific progress.

The Right to Life

I believe that the very practice of raising animals in confined environments, subjecting them to atrocious feeding habits, and killing them in inhumane ways in order to harvest their flesh and turn a profit, is a truly outrageous form of cruelty. I believe that in any advanced society, such practices are barbaric. When people ask me "What about the human body's need for protein?", I explain that if we don't switch to plant sources of protein, we'll never have enough land to feed the world. For example, producing spirulina takes 1/100th of the acreage that is needed to generate an equivalent amount of digestible protein in the form of cattle. It is notable that spirulina has twelve times more protein than beef. As these statistics show, raising cattle as the source of our protein is inefficient.[3]

I could never return to eating the flesh of an animal, and I've now been a vegetarian for nearly thirty years. I continue to campaign and raise awareness of the plight of all animals, be it within the meat industry, factory farming, zoos, and overseas animal welfare concerns, or among the feral cats that live within our communities.

We are in an age of modern technology and the internet is a fantastic tool for spreading the animals' message far and wide. Whenever I am capable of doing so, I will continue to sign petitions and raise

---

3   Mike Adams, "How to End cruelty to People, Animals and Nature, and Create a World without War and Environmental Destruction," *Natural News*, April 2, 2005, https://www.naturalnews.com/006319_cruelty_to_animals. html.

awareness of what really happens when humans seek to dominate the animal kingdom.

Finding My Calling

Through all of my unexpected encounters and connections with animals whilst growing up, and the insights I gained as a young person into how humanity treats and mistreats members of the animal kingdom, I was laying the groundwork for what would become my life's mission and vocation. The most significant event in my development, however, was my first experience of healing an animal—of connecting on an energetic soul level with another creature and restoring health and life. That story is next.

2

Timmy

W hat on earth are you doing with that cat?" was a sentence I heard almost every day as a child from my parents. I was sharing something so natural and pure: healing, compassion, and love. I owe so much to Timmy, the furred soul who helped me realize my healing potential some forty years ago. As I look back, the fact is that I owe my whole life to "that cat," as I shall explain later.

I was five or six years old when Dad bought home the scrawny black semi-feral cat to keep me company. My parents thought I needed a companion, and I did. As mentioned, I was a solitary and quite lonely child. My father worked at a Sheffield steel works, building casts, and his work colleague had taken on the task of feeding all the foundry cats. All these cats were strays that had been cast aside by uncaring owners into the harsh, industrial steel city, and through lack of human compassion, love, and adequate care, they had become semi-feral.

Timmy's Tumor

The little black cat made quite an impression on my dad. He tried to coax the tiny furred bundle to eat, but his appetite was poor. However, after a few weeks of building up trust, Dad managed to trap "Timmy" and bring the skinny kitty home.

As soon as he lifted up the cat carrier basket, Timmy meowed at me in an odd way, and I guessed it was his "special" greeting. I was immediately smitten, and overjoyed to have a soul companion to share special moments and secrets with. We bonded straight away. However, after about a week we had to take Timmy to see the vet. His appetite had decreased despite all our best efforts to persuade him to eat, and he was drastically losing weight. He was admitted to the clinic, and after numerous tests over the following days, Timmy was diagnosed with a renal tumor. The vet showed Dad and me the X-ray as he explained that the tumor was the size of a small orange. Timmy was injected with painkillers and was prescribed a course of medication to help make his cancer as pain-free as possible. We were told that the poor life Timmy had endured until now had most likely contributed to his cancer, and we were advised that Timmy would live possibly no more than one or two months. The vet requested to see him four weeks later and explained that we would need to decide what to do; I knew this decision meant having Timmy put to sleep.

Back home I was devastated. How could I allow my little friend to suffe; what could I possibly do to help him? I couldn't just leave him to die, could I?

The Healing Light

That evening, unaware of what I was doing or why I needed to do it, I laid Timmy in his basket beside the warmth of the open fire and sat beside him. I placed my hands upon my frail cat and looked deep into his sunken eyes. After a few minutes I began to feel immense, pulsating energy flow throughout the whole of my body; I felt as if I was physically merging my body with Timmy's. Then I experienced an overwhelming wave of pure love. As I stroked Timmy, his body became intensely hot as a buzzing sensation spread throughout my hands; I felt as though a light switch had turned on inside of me. Mum looked over at me, and I knew she thought what I was doing was strange, but for me this connection with Timmy felt so natural. I lightly moved my hands over Timmy's tiny body, allowing our union to be magnetized with this intensive, magical, loving energy. My hands lay there for around fifteen minutes, and Timmy looked serene and at peace. "What on earth she does with that cat I will never know," said Mum.

The Vanishing

Every day after school I'd run home, hang up my school bag, and give healing to Timmy. I told my friends about it, but they didn't understand and thought I was just that "weird kid." I couldn't wait to share the deep connection with him day after day. After about a week, Timmy started to pick up. He'd raise his head in interest at food, and he even started to eat three full meals daily. He began to play with pieces of string that I'd pull across the floor for him, and after three weeks he started to behave like a normal, healthy feline! I was overjoyed and we continued to relish our special healing connection every single day.

Four weeks passed and we took Timmy back to see the vet. As he prodded and poked my little friend, the vet had quite a perplexed look upon his face. "I'd like to run a couple more tests," he said. We took Timmy home and after a few days we received, by telephone, the results of the additional tests. We listened to a rather bemused vet on the other end of the line as he spoke about Timmy's renal tumor. The vet told us the tumor had reduced dramatically in size and, unbelievably, the growth was now the size of a pea. How could this be possible? The vet said he hadn't seen anything like it and couldn't offer us a firm explanation. Was it the healing that I'd been giving Timmy? Was it the pain-relieving medication?

To this day I can't honestly say, and neither could anyone at that time. One thing I can say is that I had the pleasure of sharing another seven or eight years with Timmy, as he passed to Rainbow Bridge aged around sixteen, peacefully, with dignity and knowing he was loved.

Timmy's Guiding Light

From that initial healing connection with my scrawny black cat, I have been guided by Timmy every step of the way, and he has pushed me on to share my knowledge of healing and communicating with animals with the hundreds of individuals who have entered the doors of my training school. Little did I know that my journey of working with animals would be one that would span many years and see me give new life to a vast number of creatures, each one having their own special place within my heart. My remarkable journey has enabled me to make many personal discoveries and acquire deep and profound wisdom from them that I will treasure forever.

All of my animal communication experiences, from my first connections on the way to nursery school at the age of four to my experience sending healing energy at the age of six, have enabled me to develop professional training courses that allow others to follow their own path in healing animals. Timmy was undoubtedly the catalyst for my journey into holistic animal therapy. He awakened the healing potential within me, showed me the way in which to put it into practice, and has walked with me at each step. We all possess the great fire of healing, and we need to become aware of how to ignite it.

A Life Saved—Thank You, Timmy

In a twist of fate, about four years after Timmy had recovered from the tumor, he returned his gratitude to me for helping him by saving *my* life and the lives of my parents.

One cold and dreary October night in the late 1970s, I felt a sweep of a cat's paw brush over my face. I was tucked up in bed and thought I was dreaming, until I started to cough. The soft brush developed into a firm tap, along with a very loud meow. I began to feel a little dizzy and then I found I was wheezing and gasping for air. As I opened my eyes I saw a gray mist swirling around my bed and realized that the mist was actually thick smoke that was permeating the whole of my bedroom. Timmy jumped off my bed and frantically wailed and scratched at my bedroom door, asking for me to open it.

I stepped out from beneath my blankets and became disoriented as I opened the door and was met by thick black smoke. It had engulfed the whole of the landing, and I couldn't see my way through. Furthermore, I failed to see Timmy. I staggered into my parents' room and tried to rouse them. Hearing my cat shrieking on the stairs, I knew he was in distress. As I was screaming as loud as I could, my parents awoke and started to cough and splutter. By now the whole of the upstairs was full of acrid smoke.

We all made our way downstairs and I scooped Timmy into my arms. We had no time to find our coats or put on shoes, so we stepped out barefoot onto the cold, wet concrete. Hearing a commotion, we walked round to the front of the house, looked up, and saw the whole of the first floor of the house next door engulfed in flames, with a man banging on the upstairs window shouting in sheer panic. I grasped Timmy tightly but he started to wriggle in fear at the noise, and then leapt from my arms to run off down the driveway. Standing on the wet earth, I was consumed with fear as my dad made his way into the neighbors' garden, yelling at the man to smash the window and jump.

"Jump," Dad called out, "smash the window." With an almighty bang, a chair landed on the front lawn along with broken glass from the window and other bits of debris, including a pair of curtains and smashed ornaments. The man was reluctant to let go of the shattered window frame, but with more coaxing from Dad, he let out a scream and leapt. He landed straight on Dad's foot! Dad was in agony, but he tried not to let it show as he ensured the man was okay.

I couldn't see Timmy and I became even more scared as other neighbors started to gather around the blazing house; luckily someone had called the fire brigade. The commotion progressed at the arrival of the firemen, but finally I could see the flames being extinguished, and the aroma of acrid smoke filled the air.

An ambulance then arrived on the scene and took the man to hospital, along with Dad, as it was concluded that Dad had suffered a broken foot. Mum and I were taken into a neighbor's house so that a fire officer could ask us questions about the event. The officer informed us that our house was unsafe to return to, and said that if we'd slept for another minute, the smoke inhalation could have killed us all.

Perhaps the most extraordinary part of this event was that Timmy had never been allowed to sleep indoors at night. Somehow he must have sneaked back into the house after Dad had put him out. Timmy saved all our lives, and for this I will be eternally grateful.

3

Awakening

The 10th of June, 1995, was meant to be a happy celebration, as it was the day of my first wedding anniversary. However, it became a memorable event for all the wrong reasons, because at the age of twenty-four, I suffered a stroke.

The neurologist concluded that the stroke was probably stress-related, as I was healthy in every other way. Warned that I would have another stroke if I dared to refuse orthodox medication, my natural, strong-willed nature nevertheless steered me to look at other methods of bringing myself back to wellness: namely, holistic healing rather than relying on prescription drugs. I chose to journey back to health without medication.

I knew my recovery was going to be a lengthy process, but it was a journey that I had to take alone. It had dawned on me that most of my stress came from the outside, from other people, so I retreated inwards. I preferred to spend much of my time alone except for the company of animals, especially my rescue cat, Sophie. The time in recovery allowed me to view all areas of my life objectively. Upon reflection, my recovery can only be likened to a death—the death of my old self—that led me to a brand-new awakening, one focused on healing myself, others, and animals.

Healing Animals

So, for over twenty-three years I've been healing animals. Along with domestic pets and livestock, I've treated llamas and alpacas, snakes, camels, and even a marmoset monkey through my system of hands-on healing, Animal Magic©. My reputation as an animal healer grew quickly from the beginning, and others wanted to apply holistic healing to their own animals. In 1997, I wrote and developed the first professional animal healer training course available in the UK, one that offered animal healing as a professional qualification and training in hands-on healing that was recognized and accepted by insurance standards, enabling graduates to work professionally. Because of its unique nature, it took a few years for the course to become approved. In 2010, I was awarded training school status for my dedication to providing quality professional training in holistic animal health care. In 2012, another unique animal therapy modality I'd developed received a legal trademark: Arbor Essentia™ (called Animal Essentia when applied solely to animals). I now teach this approach up to the master level; there is only one other Arbor Essentia practitioner worldwide. I offer some of the only diploma-grade courses in animal healing available in the UK, including distance-learning options. Additionally, I offer a course in animal herbalism called AniScentia (it shares the name of my canine herbal wellness and nutrition company), which is a more biologically based modality for natural (herbal and plant-based) healing. In 2016 I graduated as a Master Herbalist, and I also practice and teach aromatherapy; this course is called AniRoma.

Holistic treatment for animals has become more acceptable and trusted over recent years, and because of this I have trained vets, veterinary nurses, behaviorists, horse trainers, well-known people within the media, and even GPs. I have had the pleasure of teaching diverse individuals from around the globe, all with one shared passion: animal well-being. Many of my graduates now work within veterinary practices throughout the world.

I've walked my personal path through many trials in life, and animals have always found me at the crucial low moments, often launching themselves into my life. There were those in need of rescue, some that needed healing, others that required understanding, and many that lived in fear and torment. All of these connections added something extra special to my life, be it guidance, wisdom, or kinship.

Pets continue to be ever-popular in our society, yet the reasons we share our lives with them is changing. No longer are our dogs, cats, and horses "working" for their keep; they have become trusted companions and family members. They enjoy the comforts of our homes, and in recent years the benefits of improved veterinary and complementary, holistic health care.

The Holistic Animal

Holistic animal therapy, as I mentioned in the introduction, looks at the *whole* animal, not just isolated parts. It focuses on resolving the cause of the problem, not just alleviating symptoms. Overall improvement in the quality of life of the animal is the goal. Some of the therapy modalities that I will discuss in this book include hands-on healing though my Animal Magic healing system, Reiki healing, Arbor Essentia and Bach flower remedies (tree and flower essences, respectively), crystal therapy, and animal communication.

A major key in holistic care is that as a professional therapist, I look at the bigger picture of an animal's health and well-being. I compile in great detail all the information given to me by an animal's owner, with the background of the animal and their medical history being just one part of it. I look at the environment the animal came from and where it is now in relation to this, any recurrent problems and behavioral patterns, and the pet's relationship with its owner and other family members. From this information I can, along with the owner, work to pinpoint causes and develop an appropriate and feasible treatment plan for recovery and wellness. The plan may include one or several approaches, but optimum health is our main goal.

It is my heartfelt wish for everyone to begin to understand, interpret, and heal the energy emanating from our animal friends, and to tap into its richness and purity. Connecting with animals isn't just about taking them for a ride or a walk, feeding them, or praising them when they perform tricks; it goes much deeper than this. All animals share an unencumbered and enlightened energy with us. The natural vibration of animals encompasses unconditional love; their spirit is untainted, and this teaches us how we too can live in purity, with compassion and integrity. When healing is offered to them, animals accept, graciously.

Animals have no preconceived ideas about how holistic healing will integrate into their lives; they merely accept the healing offered with openness and with gratitude. They do not judge our intentions or try to pick apart how the energy works; neither are they ungrateful for our efforts. Animals intrinsically know that being part of the loving energy of healing holds the key to a deeper connection with the provider. Moreover, if the healing comes from the ones that love and understand them, greater achievements can be made. Through an animal's ability to be open to us and to healing love comes a feeling of closeness and comfort; this is empathy at its very best.

The UK has progressed greatly in recent years, and animal healing and related holistic therapy is at the forefront of the lives of many animals. Let me emphasize again that natural healing is not an alternative to veterinary treatment, but holistic approaches are totally compatible with orthodox medicine. I have witnessed miraculous results through combined efforts.

Achieving Your Dream

I am humbled by the many people who undertake training with me, especially when I hear a few months after they graduate from my program that they have decided to move away from their professional jobs to become full-time animal healers, like me. People attend training from all walks of life, including individuals who have developed successful careers in areas that couldn't be more different from animal healing. One such professional was a police inspector.

I believe that anyone with an open heart and mind can achieve great things within the realm of animal healing. I was not born with a special "gift," nor was I born into a family of healers or gifted physicians. I was incarnated into an ordinary body, and have not been without many personal trials and tribulations. Through all of this adversity and hardship, the one thing that has not diminished is my link with the animal kingdom. Sending and receiving loving energy with animals, and interpreting the healing message, is something that can be learned by anyone who attempts it with a pure heart and open mind. You need not possess a "gift"; we *all* have the gift if we just tap into a part of ourselves that has lain dormant for too long.

Healing is a reawakening of mind; it's about learning to trust our own spirit and being grateful for our intuition. It is believing that great things are possible. And they are possible; I have seen some near miracles in my work since I first helped heal Timmy nearly forty years ago.

My aim in writing this book is to share with the reader the many facets of holistic health care for animals and unravel the mystery surrounding animal healing in general. Through many years of personal experience and the hundreds of animals I have had the pleasure to work alongside, I offer the reader the opportunity to establish a deeper connection with, and understanding of, their animals. Doing so brings a richness that in itself heightens the well-being of both reader and animal.

4

A New Beginning

When I first started healing animals professionally, initially I treated horses and companion animals. However, word soon spread of my ability to help heal all species after I was featured on BBC Radio Sheffield in 2006. I was interviewed by Rony Robinson, an iconic and well-respected writer and radio presenter. Whilst on air, the show received a huge number of emails and telephone calls in relation to my interview, and I soon saw my diary swell to cover sessions treating chickens, llamas, alpacas, snakes, lizards, and even a marmoset monkey! You could say afterwards that my schedule started to get a little crazy. My reputation for being instrumental in so many animal recoveries grew, and I found that my contact information was being passed further afield—not just within Yorkshire, but in other counties too. Two interviews for BBC Radio Nottingham followed, which developed into my own question-and-answer session in which listeners would phone in with a question relating to holistic animal health.

I was then interviewed by the national press and for many animal-related publications, including *Your Cat* magazine, who compiled a very interesting feature all about my work. *The Sun* newspaper labeled me "the Kitty Whisperer," and since then I have been called a "Spiritual Animal Master," "the Animal's Magic Whisperer," "the Animal Guru," "an Animal Visionary," and even "Mrs. Doolittle" by one publication. However, I am just *me*, doing something that I was born to do, something I love: healing animals.

Throughout my years as an animal therapist, I have traveled from rural farms to city apartments, treating a wide range of animals. When I first started I didn't even have a business card, but I soon found I was working full-time as an animal healer. I was even lucky enough to be invited to treat four llamas and three dogs on an all-expenses-paid, week-long visit to a wonderful rural retreat in the Cotswolds.

I developed my training school, and my animal healing practice continued to grow through the many people who required my help and those who attended training from all over the globe, along with those who ventured into home study. However, something was missing from my own life. As well as giving healing to animal clients, I wanted to be surrounded by nature, by wildlife, and I was about to take my life to a whole new level.

A New Beginning

It was 2010 and springtime was almost upon us; a time of new beginnings, fresh growth, and a brand-new chapter in my life. Along with my fiancé, Louis, I was leaving behind all I knew—family, good friends, and a large client base—to move to Norfolk, a county one hundred and twenty miles away. We made the brave decision to relocate to this rural county just two weeks prior to actually moving. Some people said we were silly to move so quickly and give up our familiar life in Yorkshire, but we longed to live in the countryside and be surrounded by nature and all it had to offer.

Ever since I was a little girl, Norfolk has held a special place in my heart. I spent many happy childhood holidays on the North Norfolk Coast: crabbing at Wells-next-the-Sea, building the biggest sand castles on Cromer Beach, and seal-watching at Blakeney Point. One of my earliest memories of Norfolk was sitting on the steps of our holiday caravan eating a punnet of strawberries, watching wild rabbits scamper over to me to devour my strawberry tops. I was aged around three at the time. We were now leaving behind the hills and dales of Yorkshire and embarking upon a new life, one that I had dreamed of since childhood, in this low-lying county in the east of England.

Nature is abundant in Norfolk. It's a relatively unspoilt county, having few major road networks or motorways and being somewhat cut off from the rest of the UK. There's a saying that one never passes through Norfolk on the way to anywhere; you have to be going to Norfolk because you are going there! The county boasts a wonderful coastline to the north with many nature reserves. The rich diversity of the Brecks, where I now live, is one of the greatest natural areas of Britain and home to many unique and distinctive birds, plants, and animals.

With this move, I was entering a new phase. I was leaving behind a large client base of both human and animal clients and venturing into personal and financial instability; this filled me with dread. Some people said how insane we were to do such a thing, especially in such times of financial uncertainty, but it was a long-held dream, and sometimes you have to allow dreams to become reality...

In 2008, Louis's brother, John, passed away, aged just fifty-seven, from terminal cancer. Two years prior to that, I had bid sad farewells at the funerals of two of my cousins, who were aged just thirty-seven and forty-one. These emotional events had left Louis and me asking a lot of inner questions about our own lives and our hopes and dreams. We knew that we needed to take measures to achieve our hearts' desire.

As we packed the last of our belongings into the removals truck, it dawned on me that we would never see our Victorian red-brick terraced house again. Within those four walls we had shared many happy times, but we had also experienced some testing ones. The deaths of

Louis's parents, Shelia and Tom, who'd died within a year of each other; lengthy divorces for both Louis and myself, which seemed to go on forever; and a near-fatal car crash on my thirty-sixth birthday.

For the last time, I looked at my reflection in the lovely old Victorian mirror hanging in the living room. I turned the lock and popped the keys through the letterbox; the end of an era. Tears rolled down my cheeks as we drove away to our new life. My cautious Capricorn side started to kick in. I began to wonder if we were doing the right thing. Were we mad to give up our jobs, our home, and our security—everything—in search of our dream?

Jemima, our twelve-year-old ginger-and-white cat, began to vomit, breaking my thoughts of doubt. Jemima was secured in a cat carrier on the back seat of our car. I knew she had picked up on my pessimistic thought patterns. Jemima had come to live with us at the age of seven, five years previously, along with Tess-cat, also aged seven.

Our friend James drove our removals truck onwards towards the new beginning. James and his wife, Anna, were such good, supportive friends, but even with their support our relocation proved unstable in other areas, such as employment. It began to hit us that we had no home of our own to go to once we arrived in Norfolk, and that all our belongings were going into storage. For an agreed three months' duration, we would be living in a tiny two-bedroomed, mid-terraced cottage belonging to Anna and James, along with Anna's two cats Olli and Nellie, our two cats Tess and Jemima, and our dog Saskia.

Arriving in Norfolk and feeling emotionally drained, we waved goodbye to most of our belongings at the storage facility. The moving day was the most tiring day of my life. For the next three months we needed to survive on the bare essentials, and Tess and Jemima would be confined to a ten-foot-square bedroom which would be their home. It was not the easiest of transitions, at least not for the first two weeks. We were mindful of doors being kept closed so the resident cats would not come to blows with the invasion of our newcomers. Within those twelve weeks we experienced tears, apprehension, tension, anxiety, financial loss, and too much worry to mention.

Starting my business as an Animal Healer from scratch in a new county wasn't going to be easy, so we decided to take the following week to allow ourselves to settle into Norfolk life. However, fate intervened the very next day, as I received a call from a local woman named Helena who was desperate to find an answer to her dog Tinker Top's withdrawn behavior. We arranged an appointment and I looked forward to my very first animal healing assignment in Norfolk; it was a new beginning for me and also for Tinker Top, who features later in this book.

I was grateful for the phone call from Helena at that time, and previously for the opportunity to speak about animal healing and its many benefits on national radio and in the national press, as this had helped to broaden my reputation and lead me to my very first assignment in Norfolk.

5

Many Lives, One Soul

There's a vein that constantly runs through many of my students' personal stories. I hear time and time again how many animal healers sense that they have lived numerous lifetimes, feeling connected to the animal kingdom as their souls have evolved. You may even identify with this.

By becoming healers, we are reminded of who we really are: Love. This means compassion, acceptance, and sharing. These facets are an intrinsic essence of our very being. To express less than this is a choice. Maybe you feel you have always wanted to heal but couldn't explain the reason behind it? Past lifetimes may offer us some sort of explanation. It is so natural to want to offer assistance to others in need, whether human or animal; it is innate within each person to care. When someone is experiencing joyful passion, all souls within their presence are positively affected. It is a person's divine nature, their soul, which shares freely with other souls, and animals share their soul freely with us.

If, on the other hand, you have held back your desire to heal, you may identify with some of the areas below:

- Where am I holding back my love?

- What causes me to stop the natural flow of joy?

- Who prevents me from expressing my passionate nature?

- Do I permit anything or anyone to interfere with my true loving expression?

- Can I accept my own divine nature?

- As spirit, do I realize my worth?

- Is love my true expression?

- Does joy permeate in many of my life experiences?

- Is my presence uplifting to others, including animals?

- Do I choose to express my positive feelings freely?

I personally believe that animal healers have come to back to earth to assist in the spiritual shift in evolution, and to help raise the vibrations of the planet. In my experience, the areas I have illustrated below are common ground for animal healers and therapists. Can you identify with them?

Do you feel:

- As if you do not belong here on earth and are somewhat challenged to "fit in"?

- That you are on a mission to help all animal-kind?

- That you are gifted with other abilities, such as possessing psychic or empathic ability?

- That you have a deep interest in spirituality, astrology, ancient civilizations, crystals, or even mythology?

I personally believe that animal healers:

- Are often born with wisdom and inner spiritual knowledge.

- Have the ability to learn rapidly when inspired or guided.

- May have visions of past lifetimes, including in mythic civilizations such as Atlantis or Mu.

- Have overcome or are going through challenging life lessons.

- Tend to have creative and inspirational ideas, writing, artwork, or even inventions.

- Feel they have spiritual energy surrounding them in everything they undertake, and are often guided by spirit in making decisions.

Furthermore, I believe natural animal empaths often:

- Have restless sleep, often interrupted by incoming energy.

- Experience ringing in their ears (many times wrongly diagnosed as tinnitus).

- Experience tingling, goose bumps, or shivers throughout their body.

- Have waves of emotion not connected with their own feelings, picking up on collective energy.

- Change eating habits or have dietary changes, and often become vegetarian or vegan.

- Experience food intolerances, sensitivity to additives, and regularly need to detoxify.

- Look much younger than their age.

- Experience synchronicities leading to guidance, teachers, and places just at the right time.

- Have sudden bursts of creativity, a desire to write, paint, or create.

- Experience strong emotions connected with planetary alignments and moon cycles, or have an inner *knowing* that something is going to happen, such as earthquakes or tremors.

- Have a deep sense of the feelings and the needs of others.

Empathic Healing—The Final Act

"I'd like you to help Clemo, my seventeen-year-old cat," came a soft female voice down the telephone. As I went through a ten-minute consultation with her guardian, Anna, I was unsure how I could help little Clemo. Clemo was a pure white, dainty cat with hyperthyroidism and terminal cancer. As the conversation progressed I discovered that Anna wasn't expecting a miracle; however, when I went to see them both two days later at a lovely farm cottage on the edge of the Peak District, more than a little miracle occurred.

It was obvious that Clemo was ill. She was terribly thin, her eyes were sunken yet somehow inquiring, but her energy, although depleted, was engaging. Anna told me that in her younger days Clemo liked to climb the apple tree and pounce on the neighbors' cat, Tommy, who'd be sitting underneath the branches. It was a fun pastime, but the same scenario happened daily and one would think Tommy would be wise to this "game"; but apparently not, and it even seemed that he enjoyed it!

It was a late summer's day in early September as we sat beneath the boughs of the apple tree, with Clemo on her special cream blanket in front of us. Anna was softly speaking to her, whilst I held out my hands. Almost instantly, calmness washed over me and I felt totally at peace; my heart felt restful and easy. Clemo lifted her tiny head and looked up at Anna and then up through the branches of the apple tree. It was then that Anna and I knew that Clemo was ready for her journey onwards.

I touched the sides of her face; Clemo purred, then lay on her side and closed her eyes. At that very moment a soft breeze rippled through the leaves and brushed over Clemo's tiny body; her spirit had left her physical being and she was now at peace.

An emotional time followed in the subsequent minutes, but Anna remarked that this was how she wanted her gorgeous snow-white companion to pass over, not on a veterinary table surrounded by scientific instruments. Clemo had passed with dignity and love, so naturally.

I have seen what can only be described as miracles with many of my animal clients when their human believed they were at death's door, but even as a competent healer with many, many years of experience, I have come to learn that we are all on a journey, both human and animal, and that death is part of life and brings with it learning, understanding, and a new rebirth.

The Magic of Animals

When I am working alongside an animal, it's like sharing the same soul. Animals mirror our energy and our body language and this can have a great impact on their own well-being. Consequently, on many occasions I have treated both owner and animal within the same session.

A quiet and relaxed mind must be the basis of deeper connection to our animal companions, and any notion that animals are lesser beings must be swept aside. Animals should be nurtured and cared for if we are to share our lives wholly with them.

Animals are in no way beneath us. They should not be persecuted in any way or used for monetary gain, or indeed suffer untimely deaths; nor should they be slaughtered for human consumption within the food chain. If you want to develop a deeper bond, then please think a while on the above sentence. It provokes great thought and stimulates compassion.

When an animal shows unconditional love for us, it can have a deep effect on our personality as human beings. Cats don't care how we look or if we've put on a few extra pounds. Dogs don't care how untidy the kitchen drawers are, and horses certainly don't care what the latest "must have" fashion accessory is. Their connection runs beyond the superficial and is deep and everlasting. We can tap into their unconditional spirit and energy simply by placing our hands upon them, sensing their energy, and becoming a part of them within the sphere of healing.

6

Interspecies Bond

Connecting with animals involves so much more than petting, grooming, rewarding, or feeding. The mere fact that you are holding this book suggests that you too wish to deepen and enhance your relationship with the animal kingdom. Connecting in a profound way strengthens the inseparable bond we already have with our animal friends. For me, the deep bond enables me to understand animals better on every single level: behaviorally, emotionally, physically, and spiritually.

Here are a few examples of how, when we connect with animals, we can stimulate their well-being:

- We reassure our animals that they are loved.

- We learn to differentiate between their vocal sounds.

- We learn what they are feeling inside by watching the behavior they display on the outside.

- We discover what we can do to enhance their health and well-being and undertake any dietary adjustments.

- Any special needs they may have are brought to light.

- We understand why they don't connect to some people we invite into the home.

- We discover if they are in any pain or discomfort.

- We understand what they might be able to teach us on a personal level.

Mungo

One particular client developed an unusual bond with her cat, a link that she was totally unaware of and one that she didn't understand. This situation led her to an even bigger realization: how the connection with ourselves and our life can deeply affect the animals around us. This is her story.

I couldn't believe my eyes: a Cavalier King Charles Spaniel riding a Shetland pony! As I moved closer to the fence, I could see that the dog, Cassie, was enjoying her little ride immensely. Their owner, Shelley, held Cassie in place on horseback as she walked them around the paddock. However, it wasn't Cassie the dog or Camilla the Shetland pony I'd been booked to treat on this summer day; it was Mungo, Shelley's sixteen-year-old Siamese cat.

We entered the kitchen of the red-brick Victorian cottage and found Mungo in the throes of one of his fits—not a great welcome—as he lay across his blanket on the hearth rug. Mungo hardly knew we were there; his eyes had glazed over, his head was shaking uncontrollably, and frothy foam could be seen around his mouth. It wasn't a pretty sight to witness. Shelley began to comfort Mungo, as the fitting session lasted for around three minutes. I made myself comfortable beside him and I sensed all was not well with this little mite. Shelley began to speak and I felt an overwhelming sadness coming from her. The feeling consumed my body. I tried to pass it off and attributed it to her concerns over little Mungo, who lay in distress on the hearth rug.

Mungo was sixteen and, until eight months prior, had been an active cat. He was energetic for his years and happy to "help" with the care of Shelley's three horses and ponies. However, Mungo had recently been diagnosed with epilepsy and his fits were becoming more frequent, even though he was taking anticonvulsant medication recommended by the vet.

As we went through the consultation, Shelley explained that there had been no obvious incident that had contributed to Mungo starting to have seizures. She explained how she had arrived home from work one evening seven months before to find Mungo on the floor in what she described as a "trance" state. Even a plate of his favorite sardines couldn't bring him round.

The next morning Shelley had telephoned the vet and made an appointment for that afternoon. In the car, on the way to the vet, Mungo started to make strange noises. Shelley thought he was being sick, as he wasn't a great traveler, but as she turned around to look, she saw his whole body shaking from head to tail, and foaming at the mouth quickly followed. The vet concluded that Mungo had suffered an epileptic fit. The conclusion as to why he had looked so lethargic when Shelley arrived home from work the previous day was that this was probably the aftermath of what must have been Mungo's first epileptic seizure.

For seven months Shelley had been monitoring Mungo's fits, but it was a hard task to undertake, as she worked part-time in a local school as a teacher. He could have experienced more fits whilst Shelley was out working during the day. In the first month of Mungo being on medication, he sadly suffered nine seizures. In the second month it rose to eleven and in the third month an alarming twenty-three! This poor little kitty was taken back to the vet, who prescribed a higher dose of the medication and told Shelley to persevere a little longer. After a couple more months Shelley saw no change and was tired of seeing her little companion suffering, and decided enough was enough. She initially approached me whilst I was giving a talk on "Holistic Health for Pets" at a complementary health information gathering in Cambridgeshire, and we arranged her appointment there and then.

I hoped I could help Mungo in some way, so I sat beside his frail body and rested my hands gently upon him. I felt not only a depleted energy field, but also a muddy, murky energy that I felt somehow didn't belong to him. Mungo was a very weak cat, as he had lost considerable weight, and his fur seemed unusually moist in places too. Shelley commented that Mungo seemed to have lost his zest for life. He lifted his head slightly, and it looked like it was taking him an awful lot of effort to do this.

I spoke to him softly and in reply heard a quiet and delicate purr. Shelley told me she hadn't heard him purr in a long while. As it was Mungo's first healing session, it was important to allow his body to assimilate the healing energy at the lightest level, so I avoided working too deeply. I started with a body scan, as I always do before any healing treatment, to get in tune with Mungo's energy and identify the main areas in need of healing. Body scanning involves running your hands about four to five inches above the animal's body, sensing the energy as you move down the spinal region (you'll learn more about this process in chapter 9). I moved my hands from the tip of Mungo's nose down to the tip of his tail, and as my hands passed over the top of his head, I stopped suddenly. The energy had become thick and sluggish and as though my hands were wading through treacle. The area was certainly stagnant, and its energy needed to be released from Mungo's physical body. For this type of healing, I need a crystal to assist me.

I took out a clear quartz healing wand with a single termination from my bag. "Single termination" basically means that the crystal is pointed at one end; it's the perfect tool for drawing in, clearing, and moving the energy away. I began to rotate the wand over Mungo's neck and shoulders in a clockwise motion, raising the crystal slightly away from the body in a spiral action. This gesture allows negative energy to be removed, away from the physical body and its energy field. I rotated the wand again over Mungo's head and down over his shoulders. Even with the slightest movement of my hand, Mungo was looking up at me, observing my every move. It became apparent that it was becoming easier for him to move his head and neck. As I drew the wand around his kidney area, Mungo rose to his feet and decided that he needed to get closer to the crystal energy, and he made himself comfortable on my lap. The sensation I felt from the wand was now telling me to move it back near his crown area. It was then that I felt a great magnetic field. Until this point I'd been moving the session forwards quite passively, but Mungo intuitively urged me to lay the crystal across his back. I did this and he let out a huge sigh, and as I looked over towards Shelley I saw her wipe the tears from her cheeks.

In the sixteen years Mungo had shared her life, Shelley had never seen him settle on anyone's lap. I smiled as I grounded Mungo's energy, knowing that we'd made good progress as I finished with a healing balance of restful hands over his entire body. Mungo rose from my knee, stretched, walked straight over to where Shelley was sitting, and jumped onto her lap. Shelley was very emotional, and I told her to enjoy this special moment. I still felt that Mungo was holding on to a certain energy that wasn't his. The feeling of sadness I had picked up on during my consultation with Shelley remained with me, but I couldn't figure out why.

As Shelley sat with Mungo, she said she could feel a strange sensation in her chest. I asked her to describe how she felt and she told me it was the same feeling she'd experienced when her mother passed to spirit from a brain tumor eight months previously. Suddenly it was all beginning to fit together; the pieces of the puzzle started falling into place. Shelley went into great detail and explained how she felt that she had lost a vital part of herself when her dear mother had died. She told me that after her mother had been laid to rest she found it hard to do even the slightest of things, and that the behavior of all her animals had also changed towards her. She went into detail about these changes. Her Shetland pony refused to go into her stable every evening and had started to kick at the door; Cassie the dog had taken to spending more and more time outdoors curled upon the hay bales instead of cuddled up on the sofa beside Shelley, like she had done before; and Mungo had started with his fits shortly after her mother's death too.

It became obvious that Shelley was still grieving heavily for her mum. The brain tumor had developed in a matter of weeks and she felt she hadn't been able to say a proper goodbye. Shelley had made the major decision not to attend her mother's funeral, as at that particular moment in time she couldn't accept that she would never see her mum again.

I began to explain how animals react to what's beneath the surface of their human companions. We can put on a brave face and disguise our inner feelings to friends and family, but we are not this successful when we try to hide our feelings from our animals. Whatever we are feeling on the inside will give off telltale clues on the outside, in the form of hormonal and pheromone changes. Animals can *smell* our fears, our anger, our sadness, our grief, along with our happiness. I became confident that Shelley's animals had picked up on her deep feelings of grief, along with her guilt for not being able to attend her mother's funeral.

Cassie the dog didn't know how to help Shelley deal with her grief so had preferred to stay outdoors on the hay bales, away from Shelley's despair. Camilla didn't want to be confined to her stable as she felt trapped, just like Shelley did in relation to her feelings surrounding her mum, and Mungo's epilepsy could quite possibly have started because he had picked up so much disturbance from Shelley's mind, almost like an overload. I explained how animals teach us about ourselves.

Often we have to look at certain metaphors to enable us to see clearly and bring about clarity of understanding of ourselves in relation to how our energy affects their behavior. Shelley said it all made sense to her, and that this brought about a realization of how her own emotions were affecting the animals.

Three hours had passed and many tears flowed that afternoon. Outside in the garden, I took Shelley's hand and led her to a huge, magnificent old oak tree. Its mighty branches stretched out before us and we both felt immense comfort as we stepped under its overhanging boughs. We sat down upon the cool ground and allowed ourselves to connect with the pulsing of the earth, to feel its energy, to be present in that moment, not thinking about the issues of the past nor the fears of the future. I asked Shelley to ground all of the thoughts, including any guilt over the passing of her mother. I helped her anchor in the energy of the greatest mother of all, Mother Earth. I looked over at Shelley and I could see she looked a little lighter.

In the space of six weeks I gave healing to Mungo a further three times, and in that time he experienced just two epileptic fits. At the time of this writing, Mungo is three years older, at nineteen years of age, and has had just half a dozen fits. Furthermore, shortly after my second visit Shelley was able to visit her mother's house, deal with her estate, and even bring home her mum's ashes to bury beneath the ancient and magnificent oak tree where she now feels so connected.

How Our Vibration Affects Animals

I have come to realize, throughout the course of my work, how human energy can influence an animal's well-being and behavior. Animals measure their trust in us, their communication with us, and their understanding of us by the energy that we send out. This explains why Shelley witnessed the change in her animals' behavior after her bereavement.

Thoughts

When we think a thought, we give that thought energy. Watch what happens when you have a negative thought and you're around an animal. If you're having a less-than-positive thought, first observe what happens within your own body and note the changes. Dogs in particular will sense the changes on the outside; they will smell those chemical changes your body is emitting when met with inner negativity. Furthermore, if you are depressed or sad, your tone of voice will change and will most likely lower in pitch and cadence. If you are angry your tone may be louder or more piercing; all are identifiable by our animals.

Body Language

When met with negativity and feel negative emotions, our body language also changes, as it did with Shelley. On my first visit to see Mungo, Shelley was slightly hunched over and looked like she had the weight of the world on her shoulders; her animals were responding accordingly. However, by my third visit Shelley's posture had changed, her mind had eased; she was upright and she looked so much lighter. Her animals therefore were all displaying more positive behavior.

Our body posture adapts to our thoughts. If we are depressed our shoulders may slump, our head may drop, and if we're nervous our gestures may be more jerky, not smooth and controlled. We may pace, our heart rate will change, we breathe more quickly, our blood pressure shifts, and we may even perspire; this in itself promotes a release of salt. All of these bodily changes send signals to our animals. In such instances some animals may hide, some may cower, some will walk away and not look at us, and others may appear to be providing comfort by placing their paws on us, jumping on our lap, or whimpering and whining; all of these desperate actions are intended to stop us thinking negative thoughts. All animals, just like humans, respond to negativity.

Raising Our Vibration

When I'm around animals my personal vibration is always heightened, regardless of whether I'm healing them or simply petting them. Vibration can be described as "energetic spirit" (the atmosphere or energetic aura given off by a place, situation, or person; a spiritual frequency). When we raise our personal vibration we begin to resonate at a higher frequency and things become possible that aren't possible at the other end of the scale. Furthermore, healing takes place at an amplified rate. When we work to raise our own vibration, it has the benefits of increasing our awareness of animals and how they are feeling, which in turn allows them to connect with our energy in a more productive way. This is essential when healing.

You can raise your vibration by undertaking various exercises; I do so by owning my own space, through meditation and the stilling of my mind. This helps me move away from outer, mundane concerns and connects me to my inner spirit so I can emit and surround myself with a greater frequency. I believe the energy we give off, we also absorb. Psychic ability develops on a higher vibration too, and a higher vibration brings us closer to fulfilling our soul's growth. Personally, this is what aligns me to my true self. Our true self, our own vital essence, is what animals see and sense all the time.

My heightened vibration when healing allows me to be more objective, more balanced, more focused, and more a part of the animal's world. It's a time when I am totally in sync with them. This in turn allows the healing energy to flow with ease and go to wherever it's needed most; to me, this state of being is "pure resonance."

Animal Vibration

Every animal has a beautiful energy; they see the world without all the conditioning and indoctrination that we humans have. Their souls are pure; their vibrations are unbiased. One of the reasons why they enrich our lives so much is because they live entirely in the present moment.

Unlike human beings who may think, "I wonder if I should do this tomorrow" or "things will be better when so and so happens," animals react to the present moment, and when the present is gone, they move on to the next second, and so on. This is why I am humbled by their nature to trust again after having suffered so much abuse at the hands of another human being. Healing is all about being present in that very moment. It amazes me how the dog that is abused by its owner will be open to forgiving the person a minute after the abuse has taken place. The dog will respond to his owner, perhaps crawling over to them on his belly with his tail tucked between his legs, but he will still forgive.

Ultimately, however, negative human actions and our energy will eventually take its toll on any animal, resulting in either mental upset or physical or behavioral manifestations. During the course of my healing work with animals, I see horses that stamp their feet, wind suck, or have their heads hung low. I see dogs that lick their paws obsessively or urinate inside the house, and I see cats that attack others, groom incessantly, or suffer from fur loss. We all want our animals to be well, so we ask ourselves how we can fix these problems. It is, however, important to recognize that not all physical problems are physical in origin. In fact, often the physical problems I see are the direct result of a situation that the animal's human has contributed to. Our vibrations, manifested through our thoughts and actions, totally affect our animals. If we respond with concern over their wellness, we also need to recognize that there is a link between their health and our behavior.

Mirroring

Animals mirror us; they are a direct reflection of who we are. They respond to our touch, our tone of voice, our movement, and our moods. If you have an argument at work with a colleague and come home still reeling, notice how your dog responds when you walk through the door; take a look at their body language. In short, if you are having a problem with your animal, please take time to study yourself, your situations, your life, your day, your attitude, and your vibration. Your animal's issues will more than likely resolve once you take yourself into account. If an animal is suffering from a condition, especially behavioral, then I will look at how their owner relates to and responds to the world around them.

Once we become united with ourselves we establish a deeper bond with our animals, and a new world of awareness and vibration opens. I have provided an exercise below to allow you to release any negativity and just allow you to "be."

Step by Step—Animal Magic Deepening Connection Technique

This exercise is designed to deepen your connection with the animal kingdom by sharing resonance and energy with your animal, in a place of love and connection. This is always vital before beginning any form of healing. Find a spot where you and your animal will not be disturbed.

Sit upon the floor and allow your animal to lie horizontally in front of you, on tummy or side, so that you are beside their shoulder. If you are doing this technique with a horse (you and your horse will be standing), try it post-grooming, standing slightly to the side beside your horse's point of shoulder.

With your hands on your lap or beside you, palms facing upwards, allow yourself to *feel* calm, centered, and grounded.

Take three cleansing breaths but don't exhale over your animal; turn your head to the side slightly.

Observe your animal, watch the rise and fall of its body closely, and allow your breathing to synchronize with that of the animal.

Bring your mind to the center of your forehead, and focus on an invisible eye, your third or intuitive eye.

Now gently place one hand under your animal's chin, allowing them to make a connection to you by sniffing; your palm should be fully open.

Allow your other hand to stroke the animal gently, starting around the chest area (a non-threatening area) and move along to the base of their tail. Try not to touch the tail, though, as animals can often move after this contact.

Move the hand that is closest to the rear of their body back to their shoulder point, at the side of their body in line with your heart. For about a minute maintain contact with your animal; allow them to enjoy this intimate and heartfelt connection. If you wish, you may place the hand that is closest to the front of their body over your own heart too.

Begin to notice any area that comes into view in your third eye. You may notice your animal feeling tense, twitching, feeling cold or hot or damp, or that their fur, feathers, or scales become raised or even look a different color.

Begin to notice anything else and pay attention to the feelings within your own body.

After a few moments, about two inches above your animal, move one of your hands over the animal without touching the skin, from head to tail.

When you move your hands over certain areas of the body, notice again what you feel: Has your animal's breathing pattern changed? Is your animal looking around at your hands? Do you feel emotional when you move your hands over a certain area?

Are you receiving any images in your mind's eye? Are you experiencing any physical symptoms?

After around five minutes, allow your energy connection to ease and run your hands from the top of your animal's head down to their tail. Repeat this three times. This is a grounding-of-energy technique (more about this can be found at the end of chapter 9).

Take three grounding breaths and place your hands together at your heart center, as if in a prayer position.

Make notes of any connection discoveries in a journal.

This technique, if practiced a few times every week, will allow you to synchronize with your animal and to make great discoveries about their health, along with their physical and emotional well-being. Not only will you be able to ascertain any changes, it will also allow you to establish any additional emotional requirements that your animal may have. To deepen relationships with our animals when they are relaxed and healthy will help us become more aware of their "normal" demeanor. Not only will we be able to notice physical changes before they become more serious, but we will be better able to judge the effectiveness of our intuitive connection to them. Additionally, your animal will be more familiar with *your* energy and recognize it as something they enjoy and feel safe with, and will be more welcoming to your intervention should they become ill or are injured.

7

Healing Is Love

No matter what we have experienced in our lives, tucked within each and every one of us is love. To me, healing is defined as a *pure loving connection*; it's as simple as that. To demonstrate healing is to give love, unconditionally. Love is healing, healing is love. Healing is pure, without any conditions, without judgments, without restraint, and without ego.

Healing is always given from the highest spiritual and/or earthly sources. I'm a Druid, and I find that applying the twin energies of earth and spirit when healing animals imparts a channel of purity and divine connection.

Everyone Can Heal

In relation to grounding, animals who may have issues with trust and stability or those who are "highly strung" can benefit from spiritual and earthly energy combined. Animals have a natural connection to the earth, most being quadrupeds. Applying the healing energies of the earth by working as an animal healer is not reserved for Druids only, of course, nor is it limited to just the chosen few or gifted souls. The healing power of both earthly and spiritual energy are available to all, and this includes YOU! Holistic healing involves working with *all* the tools of Mother Nature, just as our ancestors did.

The Purity of Healing

When I made my first discovery about being a channel for healing energy at the age of six with my cat, Timmy, I did not know at this young age where the healing energy came from. But I became aware that when I connected to Timmy, there was an additional energy surrounding us. More importantly, I knew Timmy felt our kinship deepen, which is possibly the reason for his miraculous recovery. Just like I discovered at age six, many children can heal, and they can develop these skills by bringing them into adulthood, even if they have lain dormant for a good few years between. Anyone who has spent time around small children has seen firsthand the affinity they have with animals and how this is reciprocated.

There are many children who can heal, and I believe these special young souls will go on to create great positivity in our world. Because children don't have the preconceived ideas about energy that we adults do, they are often a purer channel for healing energy. Animals sense this and connect with children in a different way than they do with adults. Often throughout childhood we are taught to experience only the things our parents wish us to experience, and childhood can become structured and rigid, moving children away from their inner experiences that form their unique and individual personalities. To be able to open ourselves up to become a healing channel, we have to capture the essence of innocence, draw on our inner-child resources, and escape to that magical kingdom beyond the physical realm that all children are capable of experiencing.

Left Brain-Right Brain

A healer generally approaches healing from a right-brain perspective. Ever since the scientific theory positing that the two sides of the brain function differently entered popular culture, people have tended to feel a kinship with one side or the other: the right hemisphere being where intuition and creative visualization originate, the left being the domain of verbal thinking and critical analysis. Although the hemispheres work together, it's important when doing healing work to open yourself to right-brain energies, since the left brain may raise skeptical thoughts about the process. In holistic healing, there is little room for analytical energy; we must simply trust that the healing is working how it's intended to work.

For a large part of my life I relied on my left-brain traits, and even more so after working within the realm of psychology. While it didn't turn out to be my vocation, the job did teach me a great deal about myself, my life, and how I relate to the people around me and they to me. It also made me question my ability to heal animals, even though I'd seen the proof of my many achievements with my own eyes. In fact, my left-brain analytical traits began to take over in many areas of my life. I began to question my early experiences of healing Timmy and whether it was just a figment of my childhood imagination. Maybe his tumor would have shrunk anyway? Had I imagined it? At one stage in my late twenties I almost gave in to my own doubts and the opinions of healing expressed by others, especially at times when I heard people ask, "What makes you think you're so special that you can heal?" I knew I wasn't at all special, so I did question many aspects of my ability.

However, after a great deal of thought, and of course my personal experience of self-healing after the stroke, in my heart I knew that this was an innate ability in everyone. This level of being and understanding was something that our ancestors were able to demonstrate freely, but it has become lost in the progression of modern medicine. I know now that anyone can heal, if only their hearts and minds are open. Any person can demonstrate healing with another being. However, what healing actually means can differ from person to person.

How Healing Works

When I teach my Animal Magic training courses, one of the first things I impress upon my students is to not try to understand how healing works. The fact is that nobody really knows. We learn to accept that it has a profound effect on the human and animal body when we are a part of this exchange of energy, nothing more. This exchange can become miraculous, and throughout my time as a professional animal healer I have seen near miracles, echoed by many of my students with their animal clients.

The Healing Balance

Healing is all about balance: applying energy in order to balance the whole being. A whole being, whether animal or human, has many different aspects, and allowing healing to take place on the emotional, physical, mental, and spiritual levels can be as easy or as complicated as you wish to make it.

When I am working with an animal client, no two healing sessions are the same. I treat each session individually and each client holistically. The holistic approach to hands-on healing means that I treat the animal as a whole rather than focusing on one specific problem area, such as a physical symptom, given that physical symptoms can often be due to imbalances on emotional levels.

When I speak of balancing or "rebalancing" energy, I refer to the readjustment of excessive or depleted energy in a specific area or areas. It is common for subtle energy centers (chakras) within and outside of the body to be unbalanced. Energy is required for the body to perform certain tasks, such as walking, eating, and thinking, so extra energy needs to go to the various areas of the body where it is required at an appropriate point in time. (Within the Animal Magic system, I formulated Ikin, a unique method of applying healing through the colored energetic bands of the physical body. These colored bands are related to chakra colors, but are extended through meridian areas, which you apply the healing to.)

For example, if an animal is faced with danger, they need to be able to react very quickly and run away as fast as possible, or react in any other way to save themselves from the threat. In this situation, the animal utilizes energy from many areas, but the main areas are their adrenal glands (to release adrenaline), their heart (to give them the ability to pump blood faster in order to move quickly), and their head (to provide quick thinking). When faced with danger, the animal needs to be able to create an excess of energy. However, excessive energetic imbalances, particularly over the longer term, can cause emotional and behavioral distress along with physical illnesses. When healing is given to an animal, the aim is to help the body to rebalance and repair itself. Healing is a natural way of bringing the energy of the body back into harmony, but it should never be used as an alternative to veterinary treatment.

Soul Friend

To illustrate an imbalance of energy, I call to mind a client I communicated with many years ago. This particular client was healthy and well in all areas except one. It was August 1999 and I had been booked to communicate with a horse called Bobbin, a beautiful Welsh Cob, by his owner, Elaine. Bobbin lived on a smallholding overlooking Lathkill Dale in the Peak District. Sadly he had become lethargic since being rehomed from Devon three months previously. On the outside it didn't show; Bobbin was a handsome boy who exhibited an air of authority and genteel refinement.

When I communicate with an animal, I link directly to their etheric energy body through touch and/or telepathic connection (I often stand two feet away, my hands pointed toward specific chakras). This linkage enables me to tap into an animal's life force, allowing their personal story to unfold. Through connecting in this way I am able to detect any areas of imbalances within their energy spheres that may be manifesting as emotional or physical symptoms. Communicating with the animal also provides me with many answers in relation to their mental, physical, and spiritual well-being.

When I met Bobbin I took a deep, cleansing breath and placed my hands upon him, close to his heart. I felt a connection to him immediately. The words "soul friend" came into my mind. Bobbin started to snort and move his head up and down; I knew these words had connected us and that Bobbin was willing to unravel his story.

Bobbin took me on a journey where I saw in my mind's eye an Exmoor pony grazing beside a fast-flowing brook of crystal clear water. Surrounding this pony was the brightest shimmering golden trail of light. Tears started to well in my eyes, and I became emotional as I rested my hands upon Bobbin's butterfly chakra (near the shoulders; see chapter 8). He began to twitch and swish his tail uncontrollably as blue light emanated from his body and connected directly to the gorgeous Exmoor mare in my vision. Bobbin turned his head and looked into my eyes and I knew I had established the crux of his unhappiness.

For around fifty minutes I gave healing over Bobbin's broken heart. I grounded him and removed much sorrow and pain. This wonderful cob was pining for his soul friend, the Exmoor pony in my vision.

Over a cup of tea shared with Elaine afterwards, the information from our communication session struck a nerve and she immediately telephoned Bobbin's previous owner. Elaine became very emotional as she listened to the person on the other end of the line. Tears flowed down her cheeks as she heard how two weeks before Bobbin had come to live with Elaine, he had lost his soul companion, Tilly, an Exmoor pony. Tilly had contracted a neurological disease and was sadly put to sleep. It transpired that these equine partners had grazed together at the base of the flowing stream, and Tilly and Bobbin had shared an unbreakable bond. It all made sense.

Three weeks later, I received a telephone call from Elaine to say that she had offered a home to an Exmoor pony called Treacle, and how, since my visit, she had seen a positive change in Bobbin. Not only had he gained vigor and vitality, but he rushed over to greet Elaine every morning with great enthusiasm.

The Healing Vibration

When we heal or communicate with animals we tap into a sacred and vital energy source. Energy is all around us, in every living thing we see and in many things we can't. Energy is within trees and plants, in rivers, rocks, and stones. However, there are vast differences in the way each of these transmit energy. For example, the sea has a different vibration than the earth. As explorations into quantum physics suggest, everything on our planet carries its own energetic vibration and its own special frequency. It is this energy that makes complementary methods of healing such as hands-on healing, homeopathy, aromatherapy, and herbal medicine so successful; each one carries its own energetic vibration and this energy in turn connects us all. We all pulse or vibrate at different rates, but we all vibrate within the same cosmos; we are all interconnected.

It doesn't stop there. Each and every organ in the body and every illness carry a different energy too. To simplify things a little, think about the vibration of sound and how we feel uplifted when we hear a particular piece of music, or how we feel moved to tears when cutting words are spoken. Sound is a vibration, which in turn stimulates us to vibrate when we connect to our emotions. Emotions are our most powerful energy transmitters. Positive thoughts and positive emotions emit positive frequencies. When healing is applied, it can only be given with positive intent. Healing never works on a negative frequency; it is impossible for it to do so.

8

The Animal Chakra System

Chakras can be thought of as spinning vortexes of energy that carry their own unique vibration, as mentioned in the previous chapter. The term "chakra," in fact, evolved from the Sanskrit word for "wheel." The chakras are the specific locations where life force energy (prana) enters the body, and where energy circulates from. Receiving healing increases the chakras' ability to accept and hold positive energy, which helps sustain well-being. Healing balances the bodily energy among the chakras and along meridians, creating perfect harmony within the body. The chakra system provides a theoretical base for fine-tuning our healing ability.

If, for example, a cat is suffering from hyperthyroidism, the throat chakra may not be functioning correctly, as the thyroid gland is located in the throat. Similarly, if a dog has been diagnosed with hip dysplasia, then its root chakra, located near the hips and tail, may not be spinning at the correct rate.

Each chakra is associated with a particular area within the body, as each chakra is located near a major organ or gland (see chart on page 75). For example, the heart chakra is located in the middle of the chest and the solar plexus chakra is near the liver area. As centers of force, chakras can be thought of as sites where animals receive, absorb, and distribute life energy.

Energy Balancing

Through habits such as long-held physical tension, or, for an animal, their reaction to situations, chakras can amass or lose energy, and therefore become imbalanced. These imbalances may be temporary and specifically related to certain situations, for instance during house moves or divorce, or may develop into chronic imbalances, which often manifest physically in animals who have been placed in rescue centers.

When the flow of energy to a chakra is blocked or otherwise disrupted, it can lead to disease. Since an animal who has suffered some sort of trauma or abuse often does not have the ability to repair the imbalance of energy themselves, illness is the result.

Working with the animal chakras when applying healing can be an effective method of treatment. It can also be used as a preventive therapy.

Sylvy and Her Depleted Heart Chakra

To illustrate the energy disturbance within the chakra system, I'd like to tell you about Sylvy and her disfigured heart chakra.

My car was being pushed sideways as I battled against the wind and torrential rain driving along the A47. So much for it being the beginning of spring, I thought! A vehicle overtook me at a notoriously dangerous high-risk accident spot, narrowly missing an oncoming lorry. I reduced my speed as I needed to reach my next client in one piece.

It had been just six weeks since we'd arrived to start our new life in Norfolk, and here I was on my first animal healing assignment. I had been booked to treat a Welsh Cob mare named Sylvy. Since arriving at her new home, just a couple of months prior to my visit, Judy, her new owner, had become increasingly worried for Sylvy's safety. Sylvy had been rescued by Judy from a shelter in Northamptonshire; she was around eight years old and the exact color of a chestnut. Judy's main concern was that Sylvy persistently jumped over the paddock fence, heading for the busy main road. What Judy couldn't understand was why Sylvy only jumped the fence when she caught a glimpse of their gardener, Geoff. Judy had even tried to increase the height of the paddock fencing, but to no avail. Sylvy was still able to jump, which often resulted in her suffering gaping leg wounds.

When Sylvy first arrived at Judy's, Judy had felt an indescribable pain in her chest as she initially touched the horse. She described it as if someone had cut her with a knife. The feeling didn't subside even as Sylvy began to settle in.

Judy asked me to communicate with Sylvy to allow her to understand her new horse a little better, and also to see whether any information about Sylvy's past could be brought to light.

I was glad that the wild weather had abated a little when I arrived at the small farm, six miles from the ancient Norfolk market town of Swaffham. As I parked my car on the driveway I caught sight of Sylvy. She certainly was a fine-looking young lady, but I sensed sadness as I watched her grazing.

Judy came running to greet me wearing a red-checked shirt and riding breeches, with a tea towel slung over one shoulder. She reminded me a little of Felicity Kendall in *The Good Life* television series. Judy removed her gloves as we shook hands and introduced ourselves. As I entered the large farmhouse kitchen it was lovely to feel the warmth from the range permeate around the room; it was a welcome relief on a cold and dreary day. Judy lifted a huge kettle off the range and made me a cup of tea as we went through the initial consultation. After around five minutes, we heard a commotion outdoors and went out to investigate.

Sylvy was again trying to bolt over the paddock fence, doing her best to escape from the farm. The gardener, Geoff, was flailing his arms all over the place, but I could see that this was causing further distress to Sylvy. Geoff had finished his gardening duties for the day due to the inclement weather conditions and was walking back to his van when Sylvy had caught sight of him and bolted. I saw the horse had a deep-seated fear in her eyes, something which would take time to uncover. She was in panic as she bucked and kicked and tried to make her way past Geoff, and it was a time of great anxiety for all of us. Judy managed to grab Sylvy's head collar and lead her back to safety, speaking to her in a calm and soothing voice. This was the fifth incident in the past two months and we both needed to understand why Sylvy kept doing this. Geoff got into his small white van and drove up the driveway, somewhat erratically.

I stood at the five-bar gate and held out my arms in the direction of Sylvy; my palms were open and welcoming. After around two minutes the gorgeous cob engaged with my energy. As she moved closer my heart became heavy with sadness. I knew instantly that her heart chakra was depleted, and stepping closer towards her I took out a selenite crystal blade and my dowsing pendulum. The pendulum I chose was made of snow quartz crystal, which is gentle and calming, and whose energy emits a peaceful, soothing vibration. It is also a crystal that provides support whilst emotional trauma is being released. Snow quartz can also help an animal to let go of overwhelming past issues—an ideal crystal to use in a situation such as this. I looked towards Judy and saw she had rather a red face and her breathing was rapid, as the whole turn of events had caused her a great deal of stress, so I held out my hand and placed a calming piece of green aventurine crystal in Judy's palm.

I hoped that Sylvy would allow me to enter her world, as we needed to make a breakthrough and identify her strange behavior. I held out my left hand towards Sylvy with the selenite resting within it, but she stood rigid. It was obvious that this horse was experiencing great fear, tension, and anxiety. Avoiding eye contact, I dowsed my pendulum over Sylvy's butterfly chakra (near the shoulders) and began to ask permission as to whether she wished to communicate with me. Despite Sylvy being edgy, I received a definite, affirmative response, so I calmly placed my pendulum back into its pouch and lightly rested my hands upon Sylvy's poll, behind her ears.

Linking in with Sylvy's energy field, I began moving my hands around the side of her tense body. I asked her a few simple questions and she gave me all the answers that I needed. Sylvy was still in shock, and I felt as though she remained transfixed by the failed escape that had taken place twenty minutes earlier. Gently resting my hand upon her butterfly chakra, I began to communicate with her; I needed to understand what had triggered Sylvy to behave in this way.

The butterfly chakra is the all-sensing chakra. You need not stand in front of a horse to access both butterfly chakra points, given the health and safety considerations. Rather, you should stand at one side of the horse and shape your hands in form of a butterfly. When our hands are placed over this chakra in this shape, it heightens our connection to the animal and allows for an energy information exchange to take place. Communicating with animals through this central energy channel gives me a deeper insight into what area of the body may be holding tension, and can help me uncover specific areas that are in need of healing.

Judy stepped back as I allowed myself to journey deeper into Sylvy. I opened the energetic pathway, which enabled me to establish the communication link, and heard the question, "Why has he come back? I don't want to be hurt again." Then I found myself being bombarded with a multitude of questions to which Sylvy wanted answers.

I should be calm, I thought to myself, but I could feel my heart racing and adrenaline pumping around my system. Sylvy stepped towards me and sniffed my palm. I placed my left hand upon her heart chakra and she shuddered and snorted. I felt her whole body quake from nose to tail, and Judy smiled. She too knew that I had made a deep connection with her unsettled horse. These subtle body movements were showing me that Sylvy was releasing a huge amount of pent-up energy; energy that was detrimental to her health and current well-being. As I moved my hands in a circular pattern around her heart chakra, she began to raise her head and drop it in a nodding motion. I allowed the energy I was channeling to travel further within Sylvy, and the pulsing coldness that I felt in my hands told me that this horse had experienced great trauma at least once in her life. Further energy changes led me to understand how this was the key to her strange behavior; around her heart and solar plexus there was stagnant energy. As I channeled healing around her chest, I saw a murky green color in my mind's eye; there was certainly a blockage in her heart chakra.

Sylvy was now ready to communicate with me. Speaking in a gentle but somewhat anxious way, she told me how she had experienced many owners. She spoke of how her first owner had abandoned her when she was around two years old, placing her in temporary care. Sylvy explained that she had enjoyed this new start, being amongst her own kind, other horses, albeit for a short time. She then articulated that she was sold to a gentleman and this was where she had experienced most of the trauma that was currently present in her body. This man had bought Sylvy to use her as part of his breeding stock. When his attempts at bringing Sylvy into foal had failed, the man became very cruel, even abusing her physically. Sylvy had been punished in numerous ways, mentally, emotionally, and physically, and hearing her words brought tears to my eyes. In addition, numerous images came into view; I saw Sylvy standing neglected in a field and I could feel her loneliness, her insecurity, and her anxiety. She told me how her next owner was a woman who had cared for her for just a few weeks. This woman had apparently witnessed Sylvy's decline, seeing her become withdrawn and emaciated in a field close to where she lived. She had broken into the field and rescued Sylvy one evening, but sadly she could not keep her so took her to a place of safety until a new home could be found.

Her new owner was, thankfully, Judy. Sylvy expressed anxiety throughout the whole of our conversation, but as she spoke about the owner who tried to breed from her, her head shook uncontrollably. She explained "the man" was still around.

Throughout the whole of the communication session I was able to build a greater picture into the state of Sylvy's physical and emotional well-being, and also about past events which had led on to her recent behavior.

As I grounded the healing energy, anchoring it into Sylvy's energy field, the selenite crystal wand absorbed the residual negativity within Sylvy's auric field and I saw the crystal change from white to a milky cream. Selenite is a high vibrational crystal which provides clarity of mind, yet it also has a grounding effect. It is said to remove any traumatic energy out of the physical body by grounding it into the earth. Using selenite, I cleansed Sylvy, ridding her of any past energetic negativity. Sylvy's negativity was so deep-rooted, if it failed to be removed it may have blocked positive vibrations and limited future feelings of joy and upliftment. I communicated with Sylvy and asked her to feel easier as I rotated the wand around her body, and I felt the torment and distress of her past experiences being left behind. However, although I tried my best to understand how this man could still be around her in a physical sense, I couldn't. Suddenly, as I brought up my wand up over her poll, the wand flew downwards and pulled me into the energy surrounding her solar plexus. This indicated to me that this man was definitely still around her. The energy in the solar plexus area relates to the past and any negativity will cling to this area. I ended the session and thanked Sylvy for trusting me enough to share all that she had with me, though I felt that we would need to have more than one meeting.

As I passed through the gate and walked down the track, Sylvy followed me all the way down from the other side of the fence; I knew she was expressing her gratitude.

We entered the farmhouse and sat beside the stove as I explained the session to Judy. She was very shocked and became emotional when she learnt of the possibility of Sylvy's suffering. I comforted her and expressed how Sylvy was safe now. Like me, Judy was a little puzzled about Sylvy expressing that the man who had caused her so much distress was still around, and said she would give it some thought.

Two weeks later it was time for my second visit. I received a warm welcome from an extremely excited Judy. She explained how a few days after my initial visit, she had been watching Sylvy and her other horse Frederick in their paddock from her kitchen window as Geoff the gardener made his way up the track beside the paddock to the shed, where all his gardening tools were kept. Geoff had to pass beside Sylvy's paddock to gain access to the shed, and Judy explained that she saw Sylvy begin to pace and stamp her hooves. Thankfully this time she didn't quite make it over the fence as Judy rushed outdoors and threw up her arms to block Sylvy's path. She just couldn't understand Sylvy's reaction to Geoff, but this latest event prompted Judy to carry out a little investigation, and she uncovered some disturbing information. A year or so before Geoff sought employment with Judy, he had purchased horses to breed from. If the breeding attempt proved unsuccessful he would abandon the poor horses in remote places in the Northamptonshire area, where he had lived until he moved to Norfolk to take up his position as a gardener and handyman with Judy. It all began to make sense as to why Sylvy behaved in this way at the sight of Geoff! With her horse's well-being a priority, Judy terminated Geoff's employment the very next day.

My communication session with Sylvy, and all of the information I had relayed, now began to make sense to both of us. Judy was astounded and I was grateful that Sylvy had trusted me enough to share such profound information about her past ordeal, which allowed Judy to make these further discoveries.

I pulled onto the driveway and Sylvy spotted me as soon as I got out of the car, trotting over to me, eagerly anticipating our next communication session. I opened my case and selected three crystals; Apache tears (also known as obsidian) was one. This is an excellent stone to release negativity and emotional stress. It allows any sorrow to be shed from the emotional auric body whilst also promoting a feeling of stability. Jade, my second choice, is a crystal of tranquillity, building self-worth, and promoting the ability to deal positively with hurtful situations. Amber was my third crystal, as it's a very gentle and comforting stone. It carries a subtle and noninvasive energy that is both soothing and calming to the nervous system. It can also bring balance to the heart and mind.

I connected with Sylvy for the final time, and it was as if a light had been illuminated within her. Where her heart center had been a murky bottle-green color before, it was now a vibrant emerald green; the color of great healing. Holding the obsidian crystal over the sacral area I could feel her root energy center immediately absorbing the crystal's energy. Circling the jade around her heart center the energy was remarkable; Sylvy let out a huge sigh and snorted. Stepping back, I channeled the amber's energy into Sylvy's solar plexus. I moved the stone up to her crown chakra, and Sylvy lifted her head majestically, holding it there for a minute or so. I could feel healing taking place on the deepest level. Using my selenite wand, I removed the last of the residual negativity surrounding her. Sylvy turned her head towards me and looked deep into my soul; this was the look of closure. She was deeply grateful for the healing and the interpretation of her feelings during our communication. We had made a great breakthrough.

Judy, leaning against the gate, wiped the tears from her eyes as she commented, "That was the most remarkable and moving thing that I

have ever seen, Niki." Through compassion, healing, and understanding, we were able to bring about a dramatic emotional release for Sylvy
and at the same time deepen Judy's connection to her wonderful equine
companion.

The Animal Chakras in Focus

When working with Sylvy, I gave healing through three main key chakra
points: the butterfly, the heart, and the solar plexus. This allowed me to
open the lines of communication in many areas.

While human beings are believed to have seven chakras, many animal healers believe that animals have eight. I first sensed this energy
while healing my cat, Tigger, at age ten; I tried to explain to my mother
about the energy I could feel between animals' shoulder points, but she
couldn't quite grasp it, so she took a photograph of me with my hands
positioned on each side of Tigger's butterfly chakra. About seven years
ago, I realized that other animal healers frequently call this energy the
"brachial" chakra.

Each chakra is constantly giving off essential energy between the
physical organs. An animal's thoughts and feelings filter down through
the chakras to their physical body. Because a physical area corresponds
with a certain chakra, when helping heal specific physical ailments during a typical session I direct the healing energy towards the relevant
chakra. So, if I am healing an irritable bowel, I place my hands upon the
sacral chakra near to where the bowel is located.

Underactive and Overactive Manifestations

Some animals are in perfect balance. However, chakras are always unbalanced if the animal is experiencing physical, emotional, or behavioral
unrest. If a chakra is too overloaded with energy to operate in a healthy
way, it becomes a dominating force in the animal's life, often having an
undesirable effect on the human companion. For instance, an animal
with an overactive fifth (throat) chakra might be extremely vocal and

bark too much, or find themselves unable to listen to commands. Or, if the throat chakra is deficient in energy, the animal may experience difficulty in communicating its basic needs; the animal may be scared of "asking" to be let outdoors for toileting, and may consequently soil the carpet. Whether underactive or overactive, a chakra is considered unbalanced. Think of a dog abandoned in a rescue center. The dog is depressed and lonely, and because of this their heart chakra is underactive and will be unbalanced. A deficient chakra needs to open, and this can only be achieved through hands-on healing; through patience and love and understanding.

The Eight Major Animal Chakras— Their Color, Location, and Anatomical Association

Chakra	Associated Color	Anatomical Association
Root	Red	Base of tail, genitals
Sacral	Orange	Lower abdomen, spleen
Solar Plexus	Yellow	Mid-spine, stomach
Heart	Green	Front center of chest, heart
Throat	Blue	Neck, throat
Third Eye	Purple	Bridge of nose near head, eyes
Crown	White	Top of head, brain
Butterfly	Silver/clear	Near shoulders; links all parts of the body

The Energy of Animal Chakras

The animal chakra system has the ability to emit energy that will appear as different colors depending on the chakra. The chakra's shape and energy intensity carries very different meanings and interpretations for each animal healer.

The colors emitted by the energy of the animal's chakra system are largely akin to the colors in the human chakra system, and have for all intents and purposes the same functions as human chakras do.

However, there are differences. Because most animals are quadrupeds, the positioning of the chakras is horizontal, not vertical as within the human body, and they can be seen as bands of energy emanating around the animal's physical body, instead of localized areas as with humans.

Chakra Sensitivity

Given an animal's natural survival instinct, they absorb much more sensory information than humans do, and consequently their energy field is generally wider than ours. Since they receive and distribute energy through the chakras individually, they are sensitive to subtle vibrations and atmospheric changes. For example, some animals become agitated before thunderstorms or earthquakes, as they are able to pick up on vibrations that humans can't perceive.[4]

The Chakras in Relation to Behavior and Health

In addition to the eight major chakras, animals have twenty-one minor (or secondary) chakras and six bud chakras. As with the butterfly chakra, the presence of these additional chakras was something I sensed as a child, but more animal healers over the past thirty-five years now also identify with them. The minor chakras feature in the following anatomical locations: muzzle, nose, ears, and tail. The bud chakras are identified at each hoof or paw and at the base of each ear.

The eight main chakras play an important role in the overall behavior of the animal, and they can be stimulated in a variety of ways. Animals often rub their bodies on trees, inanimate objects, the floor, and even people in order to activate or balance their chakras naturally.[5] As well as being located at physical organ sites within the body, chakras also have emotional, behavioral, and physical associations.

---

4   "Working with Animal Chakras," Humanity Healing Network, http://humanityhealing.net/2013/06/working-with-animal-chakras/.

5   Ibid.

The Root Chakra

Mental and Emotional Attributes:

- Grounding

- Survival instinct

- Stability

- Security

- Trust

- Courage

- Patience

Physical Manifestations:

- Aggression

- Lethargy

- Intestinal problems

- Anal problems

- Depression

- Suppressed immunity

- Spinal problems

The Sacral Chakra

Mental and Emotional Attributes:

- Obsessive behavior

- Boundary issues

- Over-emotional

- Difficulty in establishing play time and quiet time

- Aggression towards other animal species within the family

Physical Manifestations:

- Lower spinal pain

- Hip problems

- Cruciate ligaments

- Mounting

- Urinary problems

- Impaired immunity

The Solar Plexus Chakra

Mental and Emotional Attributes:

- Feelings of abandonment

- Withdrawn

- Holding on to past issues

- Fearful

- Isolation and loneliness

- No enthusiasm

Physical Manifestations:

- Digestive tract

- Stomach

- Liver

- Ulcers

- Diabetes

- Weight issues

- Adrenal problems

The Heart Chakra

Mental and Emotional Attributes:

- Separation anxiety

- Jealousy

- Over-reliant on their human

- Unwilling to interact with other animals

- Nervous

- Has difficulty in establishing pack or herd leader

Physical Manifestations:

- Heart attack

- Lung cancer

- Pneumonia

- Mammary tumor

The Throat Chakra

Mental and Emotional Attributes:

- Difficulty in personal expression

- Is bullied by other animal members of the family

- Develops addictive or destructive behavior

- Lack of trust for human beings

- Lacking in personal power

- Prefers to be solitary

Physical Manifestations:

- Excessive barking

- Teeth problems

- Animals that are prone to nipping/mouthing
- Scoliosis
- Neck problems
- Foreleg problems

The Third Eye Chakra

Mental and Emotional Attributes:

- Thinking too much/assessing the situation at a deep level
- Stares in to space/sees things you as a human being cannot see
- Displays hierarchical tendencies

Physical Manifestations:

- Brain tumor
- Strokes
- Epilepsy
- Neurological conditions
- Blindness
- Deafness
- Depression

The Crown Chakra

The crown chakra helps to assist and balance all the other chakras within the animal's body. Within an animal, there is only ever positivity associated with the crown chakra. It is rare that the crown chakra has an imbalance due to the animal's inherent make-up and evolution.

The Crown Chakra Attributes:

- Animals involved in humanitarianism service: search and rescue, PAT dogs, horses for assistance work

- Spiritual animals who are devoted to guiding their human down the right path

- Soul animals who have incarnated again to be with the same human companion

The Butterfly Chakra—The Special Sensory Chakra

As discussed earlier, unlike the seven main chakras connected to the human being, animals have an additional main one: the butterfly chakra. This is located on either side of the animal, near their shoulder point.

The butterfly chakra is the key "sensory" chakra. This means that its energy reaches way beyond our mental comprehension. It is the "all knowing, all sensing, all feeling" chakra. In short, it is an advanced psychic center. This is also the main connection point between animal and healer. Unless I am guided to do otherwise, I always connect to the butterfly chakra first. The butterfly chakra is a link that connects all of the other major chakras together. It is the key that provides access to the mood and overall sense of well-being of the whole chakra system. I sometimes find that some animals are not happy receiving healing over their heads (especially if they are new to healing) and are often more willing to accept healing given through the butterfly chakra alone, often without the need to move my hands to any other areas of their body.

For me, connecting at the butterfly chakra provides healing at soul level, and allows me to open up to new heights of consciousness, healing, and communication between myself and the animal, often bringing immense positive changes on every level of their being.

Chakra Development

The animal chakra system is generally fully developed by the age of eighteen months. This does not mean that you will be unable to give healing to foals, puppies, and kittens, or other young animals; it simply means that the information contained within the chakra system about the health and well-being of younger animal clients may be limited.

Connecting with Your Chakra Energy

When I connect to animal chakras I am fully connected to my own chakra energy. I am connected to earth, to spirit, to the animal, and to my true essence or soul core; everything is synchronized. I believe all true animal connection experiences start with the self.

The following connection technique is a starter point for all your chakra experiences. By experiencing *yourself*, you experience the present moment. Experimenting with the technique below will enable you to become much more familiar with how your own energy works, enabling you to detect any energy imbalances within yourself before this manifests on the physical level, just like with animals. The following technique will take around ten minutes.

Step by Step—Chakra Energy Connection Technique

Find a place where you will not be disturbed.

Sit straight-backed in a chair and remove your footwear.

Close your eyes and rest your palms upon your thighs with your palms facing upwards.

Breathe naturally and rhythmically; inhale through your nose and exhale through your mouth for approximately three minutes.

Now bring your focus onto the soles of your feet and allow them to "tune in" to the earth below. You may feel a pulsing sensation or a pulling, magnetic feeling beneath your feet. Allow yourself to experience this for a minute or so.

Bring your focus to your ankles and allow your mind to rest here. What can you feel?

Then bring your focus on your calves and rest your mind here. What can you feel?

Now bring your focus to your knees and rest your mind here. What can you feel?

Bring your focus to your thighs and rest your mind here. What can you feel?

Then bring your focus to your hips and rest your mind here. What can you feel?

We are now going to raise your focus throughout your upper body, activating each chakra in turn:

- Move your awareness slowly to the base of your spine, the root chakras: Visualize the color RED in this area, a swirling disc of red light.

- Move your awareness slowly up to the pit of your stomach, the sacral chakra: Visualize the color ORANGE in this area, a swirling disc of orange light.

- Move your awareness slowly up to your solar plexus chakra: Visualize the color YELLOW in this area, a swirling disc of yellow light.

- Move your awareness slowly up to your heart chakra; Visualize the color GREEN in this area, a swirling disc of green light.

- Move your awareness slowly up to your throat chakra: Visualize the color BLUE in this area, a swirling disc of blue light.

- Move your awareness up to the center of your forehead, your third eye chakra; Visualize the color PURPLE in this area, a swirling disc of purple light.

- Move your awareness slowly up to the top of your head, your crown chakra; Visualize a streaming WHITE, vibrant light entering the top of your head and flowing all the way down your torso, down your legs, through your feet, and entering the earth.

- Focus and rest at your feet for a minute or so, and when you feel ready, take a deep grounding and balancing breath.

- Allow your awareness to fall onto your physical body and open your eyes whenever you feel ready to do so.

Journaling

You may wish to make notes in a journal for detailing your experiences during this awareness connection journey. Consider the following areas for inclusion:

- Were you able to feel relaxed throughout the connection technique?

- Did your mind wander or did any thoughts reoccur in your mind?

- What sensations did you experience in your body?

- Did you feel a connection to each area of your body? If not all areas, which ones?

- When you were visualizing the colors, were you able to see them clearly or did any look murky? Were there any colors which failed to show?

- The white light; did this become stuck anywhere in your body?

- Were you able to ground yourself?

- How do you feel now?

Making personal notes will help to stimulate your right-brained capacity, linking directly to creativity and experience. You can later reflect on your experiences, and as you repeat this exercise you will become aware of how your chakra system changes and develops.

9

Animal Healing in Practice

You will now be familiar with my message throughout this book: each and every one of us is capable of healing animals. Hands-on healing—which involves body scanning, connecting with the animal, and sending healing energy through the chakras—is an invaluable therapy in keeping our animals healthy and happy. Ongoing, regular healing sessions can help restore, replenish, and maintain the natural harmony within animals, which supports their optimum health and well-being. Many people often think of using healing only when their animals are sick or injured, or when they are suffering anxiety or stress. However, healing is a wonderful way to help your animal relax and unwind, and it allows you to notice any physical or behavioral changes that may not be apparent on an everyday level. Not only can we notice these changes before they become more serious, but we are able to judge the effectiveness of giving healing and how our animals may respond in a crisis situation before it actually develops. Spending time each day, or each week, sharing healing with our pets helps us to deepen our relationships with them. Additionally, your pet will be more familiar with your personal energy during healing, recognizing it as something they enjoy and feel safe with, and so will be more receptive to that sort of intervention from you when they are ill or injured.

Are You Ready to Heal?

Through healing animals I have also healed myself. This vocation and path of my soul has allowed me to explore the many facets of my own personality, mind, and spirit, enabling me to make inner discoveries that may have remained hidden had I not followed my heart and walked the healing path. Had I stayed in the field of orthodox medicine, I would not be the person I am today.

Giving time to heal others is also about devoting time to yourself, to develop your healing ability. Universal energy is not in a state of waiting; it is always present within you. You don't have to wait for anything in order to turn to your inner dimensions for guidance. For example, many may think, "I'll begin my healing journey when my children leave school" or "when I'm more financially secure." There really is nothing to wait for; its presence is within the current moment. Healing transforms our experiences and opens us up to life as it is. It allows us to be guided by a deeper sense of belonging that can't be expressed in words. For me, healing opened up an entirely new view on everything. Give yourself some time to dive into and explore your divine nature and healing essence.

Establishing Bonds and Boundaries

There is much preparation and many areas of consideration before you begin to give healing to animals, even if you are just giving healing to your own pets. Just like humans, animals have boundaries, and if we cross these we betray their trust. Following the guidelines below should help you to maintain a healthy respect for your animal during the whole healing process. When initially approaching the animal to give healing, it is helpful if you understand them. Just like us, they have feelings of affection, fear, stress, and happiness. They send out clear signals about their feelings and have a large repertoire of body, facial, and vocal language. They understand words in our vocal language, and respond to images too, so send positive, passive, and nonthreatening thoughts to them and speak in a softened tone as you approach them.

The Ethics and Protocol of Healing Animals

Every animal health professional has a code of ethical conduct to adhere to. This code of practice helps protect the animal client and the healer from any misconduct or mishap. I have illustrated this with my own short guide to Animal Magic ethical practice:

- Never diagnose an illness; no healer is qualified to do so.

- If you suspect your animal is suffering in any way, or suspect an undiagnosed condition, then your vet must be the first point of contact.

- Always ask the animal if they want or need the healing, and observe their answer closely. This can be done in a variety of ways: telepathically, or using your intuition through pendulum dowsing/energy field testing, etc. See the chapter on the pendulum in this book.

- Recognize that healing energy is not derived from any physical power we possess as a human being; rather, the healing energy belongs to the Great Creator/God/Buddha/ the earth/the Goddess/Spirit etc.; whatever name you prefer to use. The energy only passes through us; we are a healing channel; we are not giving away or depleting our own energy resources.

- Recognize that optimal healing occurs when the animal and the healer work together towards the required state of well-being, allowing the healing to flow where it needs to go and not necessarily to the areas we want it to flow to.

- Healing energy flows to wherever it is needed most.

- Always prepare yourself before you give healing, and ensure you are in an appropriate frame of mind. Never use mind altering alcohol or drugs before, during, or after a healing session.

- Never give healing when you are feeling any negative emotions, such as anger or rage, and avoid channeling healing to another if you are feeling depressed.

- Approach each healing session with calmness, confidence, and total awareness.

- Be truthful about your healing experiences. If the animal isn't responsive, be honest.

- If you live in the UK, always work within the framework of the Veterinary Surgeons Act 1966. This act is a large document appertaining to animal practitioners in the country. It contains guidelines for nonlicensed veterinary surgeons and covers specific areas of practice. As animal healers, we are prohibited from diagnosing and providing medication. Under this act, animal healers are not allowed to give healing to an animal as a replacement for veterinary care. Be sure to research what the relevant guidelines are in your specific country.

- Respect and value orthodox medicine; any negative thoughts about other types of medicine are points of resistance. All medicine can work together harmoniously, if allowed to do so.

- Never contradict the recommendations of a veterinarian or suggest that any animal should change or reduce the prescribed medicine or treatment.

- Regularly monitor your views of your animal's health condition to be sure that you are not projecting (rather than intuitively reading) their true condition and their healing needs.

- Never violate free will by imposing energy healing on those animals who don't want it. Animals will walk away if they don't require healing, so never force them to stay.

- Do not take on the animal's disease. Your own body is sacred.

- Acknowledge that healing animals can at times be emotionally tiring. Depending on your own physical and emotional health, it may require you to rest and replenish yourself between healing treatments.

- After giving healing, always be thankful to the Great Creator and all of your helpers for each healing experience, along with giving thanks to the energy itself.

- Complete the healing process with a grounding and protection prayer and/or ritual (see page 110), so that you and the animal are fully connected with your physical bodies afterwards.

- Use your gifts of empathy and intuition, work from your heart, never with ego, and you won't go far wrong.

Animal Magic Health and Safety

You need to be aware of the elements of health and safety when working with animals, such as understanding the danger possibilities of working with feral cats or how not to get bitten when working with rescue dogs. A lot of this is common sense; however, working with horses needs additional consideration because as you become relaxed during the healing session, injury becomes a real possibility. Physical injury from a horse can be inflicted by biting, stamping, rolling, or kicking. Non-socialized horses tend to be the ones that are most aggressive due to their lack of human interaction. Such horses can be easily startled and upset, and it is more than likely if you decide to become a professional healer that it will be these souls who find their way to you most often.

When I am giving healing to a horse, I never bend down at their rear end. If the horse moves suddenly, it has the potential to knock me onto the floor and trample over me before making its escape. I also ensure I am wearing hard, protective shoes. These are a must when working with horses; no soft shoes please.

Biting is another possibility. I have only ever been bitten once by a horse and I don't think this was out of malice. The horse in question just became a little too engrossed in the healing, and when I was closing the energy link down, he reached out and took one of my fingers, then a chunk of my hair, possibly mistaking it for hay!

If you are giving a treatment to a horse for the first time, it will obviously be a new experience for both them and you. New experiences can sometimes make horses react in uncertain or unpredictable ways; ways that may be out of usual character. Always be prepared for this, and if possible have another person close by "just in case." It is almost definitely a safer option to give healing to a horse in an open area, such as a paddock, and not in a confined stable or loose box, as you can walk to safety more easily if needs be.

Bacterial contraction is possible when working with horses. Salmonella and campylobacter are two bacterial agents that can be transmitted from horses to healers. Even healthy animals can carry and spread salmonella. Transmission to healers is by fecal to oral route, so to avoid this it is imperative to wash your hands with soap and water, or an antibacterial wash, soon after the healing ends.

Caution for Clothing

In over twenty years of working as a professional animal therapist, I have also acquired additional knowledge in the preferences of the horses I treat—one of which is to be mindful of the type of clothing worn when healing horses, as they hate coats that scrunch! Waterproof coats, albeit great for inclement weather, can prove just too noisy for horses, resulting in them becoming startled. Gore-Tex and the like isn't a horse's friend! Scarves should not be worn either, for fear of your becoming strangled if its grabbed quickly by the mouth of a horse.

Smell

Be aware of how you smell. Avoid wearing perfume when you are working with animals, as they could find the smell very invasive, resulting in unpredictable behavior.

Move Slowly

Finally, always be mindful of your actions when giving healing to animals; move gently, slowly, and calmly, avoiding sudden movements. Be aware that as you read the energy of the animal, they are also reading you!

Journal Keeping

Keeping a journal to record details about your animal, the treatment you give, and your animal's reactions will help you develop your observational and practical skills. The more changes you notice, the better equipped you will be to help your animal. Whether you are addressing a specific health issue or sharing regular healing sessions, recording the initial condition of your pet, what you did during the session, and your animal's reaction will provide invaluable information later on and help you understand their behavior. This will be your guide for successful future treatments.

Healing the Individual

No two animals are alike. Animals from the same litter will display some of the same traits, but will not be exactly the same as each other; therefore, they may not respond in entirely the same way during a healing session. Environmental factors can also determine how the animal will respond during the treatment. For instance, a cat in a rescue center will respond very differently than a cat within a domestic home environment. In addition, animals that experience healing for physical ailments will react differently than those accepting healing for emotional turmoil. With this in mind, every healing session needs to be explored differently, and each healing treatment should be tailored to suit the specific needs of the animal with all of the above areas factored in. You will learn as you go; healing is a constant learning process.

Key Factors in Healing

Many people are unaware that some behavioral changes within their animal can stem from the animal being in physical pain, or because they are suffering from some emotional upset.

Changes in animal behavior that indicate pain or emotional disturbance can include:

- **Confusion or disorientation:** The animal may get lost in his own back garden, or become trapped in the corner of their field, or behind furniture. They may suddenly become unaware of their familiar surroundings.

- **Pacing and being awake all night, or a change in sleeping patterns:** Even wailing noises from cats, snorting from horses, or whimpering from dogs can all be distress signs if heard during the night or at unfamiliar times.

- **Loss of house-training ability:** A previously house-trained animal may not remember where their litter tray, the door, or the cat flap is, and may urinate or defecate where they normally would not.

- **Decreased activity level:** Your animal may become lethargic.

- **Decreased attentiveness or staring into space:** Looking lost and bewildered.

- **Not recognizing friends or family members:** Barking excessively, or rearing up at familiar people.

- **Becoming unusually aggressive or starting to bite:** Scratching or nipping familiar people.

- **Developing a sudden fear of noises:** Becoming easily startled, and trying to flee in distress.

- **Becoming fixated on one person:** Or suffering from separation anxiety, or even becoming unusually demanding.

Many behavioral changes can be due to underlying medical conditions. If your animal's behavior is changing, have them examined by your vet. With patience, understanding, veterinary treatment, and holistic healing, you can help make your animal's life one of quality which will benefit you both.

Animal Awareness

Since animals can't converse with us on a verbal level to explain how they are feeling, the following observations in relation to their past (if the animal is from a rescue center) will help you to uncover why they behave the way they do, or how they relate to people or certain situations. By identifying some of the key areas below you will become aware of what may be happening on a physical, emotional, behavioral, or even spiritual level in your animal's life.

Environmental History

- Do you know the history of your animal?

- How old was your animal when it came into your life?

- Did your animal have a previous home or shelter, or was it a stray?

- How long has the animal been with you?

- Do you and your family move house often, or have you been at the same address most of your/their life?

Physical History

- Does your animal have any known illnesses?

- Has your animal undergone any medical procedure(s) or had any injuries, especially those that did not heal too well?

- Is there any current discomfort from past medical issues?

- If there is an illness or injury that is not healing with proper veterinary care, was there anything going on in your life at or around the time the illness began, or when the injury happened, to inhibit the correct healing of the animal?

- Was there ever any abuse that you are aware of?

- What is the animal's daily routine? Are there any recent changes to this?

- When, how often, and what type of exercise does the animal receive?

- When, how often, and what type of play does the animal enjoy? Is this indoor play or outdoors?

Habitual History

- What is their family group status with other animals in the household? How about their status with the human residents in the home?

- If there is more than one person in the house, who provides the animal with food, exercise, play time, and discipline most often?

- How is the animal's appetite? Are there any recent changes in dietary requirements?

- What are their elimination habits (urinary and bowel)? Are there any recent changes?

- Have there been any recent changes in the household? Did anyone leave? Is there a new member? Have there been any lifestyle changes for anybody?

Behavioral and Emotional History

- Is your animal usually well-balanced?

- When did any "problematic" behavior start?

- Is there a logical reason for the animal to be exhibiting this behavior?

- When is this behavior at its worst? What time of day? Are there certain circumstances, specific locations, certain people, or other animals that trigger the negative behavior?

- Can you break the behavior into specific aspects? If so, which aspect is the most unacceptable to you?

- What, if anything, have you done to try and change the behavior? What was the animal's reaction?

- What is your direct reaction to the animal's behavior? Do you feel angry, frustrated, guilty, or fearful?

- In what way do you want the animal's behavior to change?

- Allow yourself to be in the animal's position. What do you think your animal might be feeling, and why? What reasons would they have to behave this way? (Intuitive answers are acceptable.)

- What was going on in your life at or around the time the animal's behavior started?

Objective Observations

- What is your animal's general demeanor? Are they alert and listening to you? Do they seem happy, anxious, energetic, tired, etc.?

- Are their eyes dull or bright? Clear, cloudy, or watery? Are their eyes able to focus easily? Do they have fur overhanging their eyes?

- Are they over or under weight?

- What is their overall muscle tone?

- What is the condition of the coat? Clean or matted? Dull, lifeless, dry, or shiny?

- Are there any bare spots on the coat? Any specific areas they have been scratching, licking, or biting?

- What is the condition of their paws and nails, or hooves?

- How are they breathing? Fast or slow? Deep or shallow? Are there any soft or loud noises on the inhalation or exhalation? Do they make a vast amount of noise when asleep?

- Is there any panting, snorting, or coughing?

- Are there any unusual odors?

- Does your animal appear to be in any pain?

- Are there any signs of a recent injury?

- Notice how the animal moves. When walking, are their movements smooth or do they show any stiffness in the joints? Do they limp or have an uneven gait? Do they prance, or jog, or walk unevenly or gingerly?

With all of the above considerations, you can begin to understand what contributes to your animal's life and how these key areas play a role in their behavioral, emotional, and physical well-being. Giving healing to an animal enhances your awareness of how the energy affects them, and on what level. I am not suggesting you interpret the level of healing that the animal is going to absorb, as it is important not to have any preconceived ideas about what may and may not be healed. I am merely suggesting that you become *attuned* with your animal, understanding their past and their present level of being, to make the healing more effective and enhance the overall process.

Connecting to the Healing Source

You may at first doubt your ability to give healing. You may not even feel particularly connected to the energy itself. It's natural to feel this way. However, practicing the following exercise technique as often as you can will enable you to establish an awareness of how your own energy can *create* energy, which in turn allows you to establish a greater connection to the energy source and will enable you to feel how healing actually works.

Step by Step—Connecting to the Vital Healing Source

Take three deep breaths to ground and center yourself. Feel your breath flowing freely from your lungs, down into your stomach, and all the way down through your body, out of the soles of your feet into the earth below.

Now place your hands together over your heart center (chest), in a prayer position.

Take another deep breath and on the exhalation allow your breath to pass over the tips of your middle fingers, allowing yourself to feel cleansed and empowered. The tips of the middle fingers are a key part in both earthly and spiritual energy

Next, place your hands on your lap, palms facing upwards, and take another three deep breaths.

Now bring your palms together in front of you and rub them together in a circular motion for about twenty seconds.

Allow yourself to notice all the sensations you are feeling: Tingling, pulsing, throbbing, heat, coolness.

Notice your energy: Is it moving outwards from your palms? Is it moving in another direction? Is the energy concentrated in the center of your palms? Is it moving into or through an area of your body? Are you experiencing anything else?

Now rub your palms together again for a few seconds, then hold them facing each other, about two inches apart, and notice the ball of energy between them. You should feel a repelling of energy, a little like the force of a magnet.

Place this ball of energy into an area of your body, your heart center, your thigh, your throat, etc., and notice any effect this has on you.

Now place your palms facing downwards on your thighs and allow any excess energy to flow into the earth below to ground you. Take a deep grounding breath.

The ball of energy in the above exercise is called "subtle energy." This is akin to the energy we experience when we apply healing.

Focusing Your Mind

Try the above connection exercise as often as you can. You also need to focus your mind and allow nothing to intrude on your thoughts. Stay in the present moment. If thoughts keep cropping up in your head, they will inhibit your energy flow and the healing session will not be as effective as it could be. Being present in the moment doesn't mean that you're not concerned about tomorrow or the future; it means focusing your attention right here and now, and feeling committed to supporting the animal's health and wellness journey.

Healing energy is created by:

- **Stilling your mind:** Concentrating on nothing but your own breath, your own body and that of the animal.

- **Grounding your body:** Breathing into and through your body, not holding on to your breath.

- **Maintaining your focus:** Being aware of your experiences and feelings and being present in that very moment.

- **Creating positive action:** Creating the energy healing ball and allowing healing to flow through your animal client.

- **Demonstrating the healing energy:** Maintaining connection with your animal and moving your hands across the body to wherever the animal or your intuition guides you.

Step by Step—Preparing to Heal

When applying any form of holistic therapy, you need to ensure your environment is conducive to the well-being you wish to stimulate. Choose an area of the home and a time when you and your animal will not be disturbed. You should both be relatively relaxed so it's a good idea to give healing a little while after the animal has eaten.

Tips for a Positive Healing Session:

- Unplug the telephone(s).

- Ensure neither you nor your animal are hungry; rumbling tummies will not be conducive to an effective session!

- Have some soft music playing.

- It is preferable to have just the animal and yourself in the healing room.

- Do not burn incense, as aromas such as this can be disturbing to an animal's highly tuned sense of smell. Do not wear perfume or strong deodorant either.

It is important to be clean in body and mind, and pure in heart. If you have had a bad day at work, or are holding a grudge for some misdemeanor, then it won't be an ideal time to connect with your animal.

Heart Consciousness

Whenever we heal, we are giving the essence of pure love. We are interweaving our true human essence with the soul of the recipient; we become one. Animals see our true soul essence every day. It matters not to them if our hair is a mess, if our clothes are stained, or if we don't have as much money in the bank as we would like. Animals see beyond all our complexities and recognize the part of our soul that is pure, especially when we are healing them. Healing an animal is a time when we can be totally free in mind, body, and spirit. It's a time of complete connection.

Integrity

Anyone who has attended one of my training courses, who has been a client of mine, or who knows me well, will tell you that I don't "do" egos. I am no better or worse than anyone else. I don't seek praise from people in power, nor do I tear myself to pieces when, on the odd occasion, an animal fails to make a complete recovery. Every experience is part of my learning process and I can only learn through being connected to myself, not through the opinions or ideas from others about how I should be, heal, or live.

If there's one piece of advice I would add to this book, it is to allow yourself the freedom not to care about other people's opinions of you. Whatever you do in life, others will base their views and thoughts on what it is they have within them. If they have a free heart and mind, they will love you even when, to them, you are wrong for wanting to be a healer; they will still guide and support you. We are all learning, and "acceptance" is a key word in the world of healing. If such people haven't freed themselves from their inner demons or their own personal blocks, they will hold against you even things you do well. This is because human nature creates the lens with which to see the world. Two people can look at the same object and see two totally different things, and have two totally different feelings and perceptions of what is in front of them. There should be no judgment within healing, just different forms of experience; don't become a prisoner of judgment.

So, become a healer, be proud of being a healer, and stay true to your heart and soul purpose. We can all recall a situation where we didn't say what we really meant, felt, or wanted, and when we lied, pretended, or acted because we felt we wouldn't fit in if we expressed how we really felt. You will then have noticed that such a situation bears heavy emotions. Therefore, never be afraid to express who you really are, because that would be deceiving your soul. Not caring for the opinions of others doesn't mean you'll always do what you like, no matter the consequences and effects on other people. It means that every choice has a responsibility that goes along with it. The universe supports those who support themselves.

Respecting Animal Connections

Every animal has their own boundaries and we should be mindful of these at all times. We should also understand that they have their own free will. Every animal is different and unique. Most animals will welcome the healing you give to them, but some may find the energy a little too invasive and you may never get to give a full hands-on healing treatment, however hard you try. Making initial friendly contact will enable your animal to become accustomed to your smell, your auric field, and your energy. All these things will help an animal build up a bigger picture about you and will bring them a step closer to accepting the healing energy on offer.

Respecting Yourself

When applying healing, you need to be fully aware of the animal and how they're processing the energy being channeled. You also need to know that your energy field (aura) will be mingling with this energy, so whatever you are feeling will be picked up by your animal. Before you begin to apply healing, you should protect your own body from picking up on any negativity the animal may be carrying. Failure to follow a basic protection technique may result in you feeling spaced out, nauseated, unbalanced, or generally out-of-sorts for a length of time after the treatment.

Step by Step—Self-Protection Method

Take a few cleansing breaths. Really feel your exhalation releasing any negativity, and your inhalation empowering, strengthening, and protecting your whole body.

Raise your awareness to your third eye area (in the center of your forehead).

Now raise your awareness further up to the top of your head.

Allow yourself to feel a protective energy moving up through the top of your head and connecting with your higher self/God/the Goddess, etc.

Allow this feeling to flow out through the top of your head, bringing the energy down over your physical body as if it were a shower of protection. Allow it to radiate and protect your physical body in a cloak of defence.

Once the energy shower has reached your feet, begin to feel empowered by its protection.

Take three deep breaths and make connection with your animal.

Making the Connection

After an initial bond has been established, it is then time to make connection with your animal. Now that you have prepared the environment and yourself for the healing session, you need to prepare your animal client.

Have your animal lie down anywhere that's comfortable for both of you. Ideally you don't want to be stretching under a table or over a stable door to reach them, nor do you want to be squashed into the corner of a paddock, putting your own health and safety at risk. If the animal wishes to sit instead of lying down, this is fine. Horses often prefer to stand during healing; this is also okay.

When I'm giving any animal healing, I like to become part of their world, physically. This means I will usually sit on the floor if I'm treating a companion animal such as a dog, cat, or rabbit; but if I'm healing a horse, I will work outdoors in a natural grazing environment instead of the confinement of a stable, loose box, or field shelter.

Explain to your animal what you are going to be doing, speaking softly whilst petting them. Even though they won't be able to fully understand every word, they will certainly understand the energy that accompanies your speech.

Does Your Animal Want Healing?

This is a question that only you will know the answer to. By being fully present, by observing their reaction when you sit at the side of them, by centering and focusing, it will give you a good indication of whether the animal is a willing participant in their healing process.

Another way of determining the response from your animal is through using a dowsing pendulum. I have used a dowsing pendulum for over twenty years within my healing practice, and it has never once let me down. There are so many differing beliefs about using dowsing pendulums. Some people believe that the answers you receive from the pendulum come directly from spirit, while others believe that answers come from your higher, intuitive self. If you do wish to use a dowsing pendulum for animal healing, then read chapter 12 in this book.

Intuitive Listening

Tell your animal you are offering healing out of love for them, and then ask them if they are happy and if there is anything that they do not like. Quietly listen and observe them, and see what images or words come into your mind. I found that Jemima, one of my cats who is now at the Rainbow Bridge, always projected colors into my mind in relation to areas where she needed healing. For instance, if her lung area was in need of healing, I would see green in my mind's eye; if her throat area needed healing, I would see the color blue.

Body Scanning

When I speak of body scanning, I'm not talking about those huge machines at the hospital, of course; I'm speaking about scanning the animal's energy field by moving the palms of your hands slowly above their body to feel any fluctuations or changes of temperature. You will generally feel fluctuations of energy in areas where emotional, physical, or mental energy has become stagnant. This stagnant energy is often called "energy blockage." Doing a body scan will bring into view any areas that may need additional healing, areas where you need to hold your hands for a longer period of time.

When Body Scanning Is Used

Body scanning can be used prior to giving an animal healing and is good for locating blocked chakras. Once these blocked areas have been detected, healing energy can be directed solely to them, and they may immediately return to their normal vibration. Long-term blocks may also begin to slowly dissipate, promoting emotional and mental repair for the animal.

The Body Scan in Practice

Many of my clients have asked me how I can tell if an animal is sick or has the initial stages of a potential health problem. One way is through doing a body scan; I simply allow my hands to move over their entire body, detecting any fluctuations in energy. I feel a variety of sensations in my fingers, my hands, or my body, dependent on the animal or the severity of the problem I'm healing. These fluctuations can range from heat, to coolness, to tingling, to dampness, etc. I may even experience these changes within areas of my own body.

If I sense a rather dramatic change in energy, I advise the client to take the animal to their vet, adding information as to where a potential problem may exist. It is important to note that this is not a veterinary diagnosis, as I am not qualified to do that; it is energy-based only. When healing one particular feline client named Chaz, I detected a problem in his sacral chakra (kidney) area. Chaz was taken to the vet, the appropriate tests were done, and it turned out that he did have mid-stages of renal failure, which if left untreated could have proved fatal. It is important to remember that body scanning is *not* a veterinary diagnosis tool. It is merely used to detect energy imbalances, enabling the healer to channel the energy towards specific bodily locations.

Step by Step—The Animal Magic Body Scanning Method

Stand or sit at the side of your animal, holding your right hand two to four inches away from the animal's body. Place your left hand over the center of their forehead or at the back of the neck, ensuring you don't touch them.

Move your right hand smoothly and steadily over their neck, down to their tail, passing slowly over the spine and paying particular attention to the overall *feel* of the animal's energy.

Do this a second time, this time even more slowly, noticing minute differences as your hands move over each area. One place may feel hotter than another, which indicates drawing in energy; another more cooler, which indicates energy flowing outwards. Perhaps the energy feels thicker or thinner as you move your hand over other areas? There may be subtleties that change from place to place.

You can now carry out a complete healing treatment with this additional information, and target specific areas.

Butterfly Healing

I nearly always place my hand on the animal's butterfly chakra to begin a healing session, my other hand resting over my heart chakra; this is soul-to-soul connection to the source of pure love. You may not always be able to connect to the butterfly chakra due to injury, soreness, or an open wound in this area. If this is the case, depending on the animal's size, stand or sit beside them and connect heart-to-heart; one hand resting on the animal's heart and one hand placed upon your own chest.

When I feel the start of the energy flow, I then place both hands upon the animal and move them to where the animal or my intuition guides me to in order to apply healing.

You should never give healing directly over an open wound. This is because you may stimulate tissue regrowth at a faster rate than desirable, causing the wound to suffer additional tissue trauma.

Observed Responses During Healing

Obvious physical reactions may include muscle spasms and twitching, curving of the spine or arching the back, licking, salivating, panting, chewing, or yawning.

Breathing more deeply, lowering their head, closing their eyes, and generally being more quiet and relaxed are signals that the animal is benefiting from your treatment.

Other more subtle reactions include changes in facial expression, such as softening of the eyes, or relaxing of the chin or ears. Even abdominal sounds might signify the release of energy; your pet may even "toot" a little, so don't be alarmed if this happens!

The animal might respond differently to specific points or areas you are healing. The more aware you are of their response, the better you can "fine-tune" your treatment to their individual needs.

Equine Observations

Horses are wonderful to work alongside. However, they are huge, powerful animals, and if we lack the confidence to work with them they will pick up on this and may try to dominate the interaction. It is imperative to understand some key areas of equine body language when applying healing or doing a communication session (remember that these are usually undertaken as separate modalities or sessions).

Observed signs of responsive equine behavior:

- Changes within their face and muzzle; frequently becoming relaxed and often with a hanging tongue

- Eyes moving to half or fully closed

- Head becoming heavier and body dropping

- Nose and nostril twitching in response to facial energy release

- Muscle flinching or popping sensations; this often indicates a change of energy within the body, commonly moving from cold to hot as you apply healing

- Licking around their lips and mouth, and possible tongue flicking

- Extending or contracting any specific muscle or muscle groups

- Swishing of tail, either side to side or backwards and forwards

- Noises indicating a release of energy or pent-up emotion; noises include neighing, sighing, or snorting

- Noticeable changes in skin temperature or the surrounding area in which you are working, even drafts appearing from nowhere

- Slower heart rate

- Looking around at your healing hands

- Yawning or stretching out the jawline

- Body looking generally relaxed

- Changes to the appearance of their hair; standing on end/fluffed or puffed out, dull, shinier

Observed Signs of Pain:

- An unwillingness to absorb any healing given; maybe flinching when you move to certain body areas

- Groaning or moaning noises

- Frequently and jerkily looking around at their body for no apparent reason

- Teeth grinding or wind sucking

- Rapid heart rate or chest palpitations

- Rearing of their head or any part of their body

- Aggressive tail-swishing

- Stamping or scraping of hooves

- Bucking or rearing

- Wrinkling of the nose

- Stiffened or flattened back ears

- Teeth and mouth looking different

- Trying to escape their stable, or bolting to the other end of the field or paddock

Post-Treatment Actions:

- Encourage your animal to be still and calm; no long walks, hacks or agility classes after (or before) a treatment!

- Ensure that water is readily available after any healing session, as animals instinctively know that water is a beneficial healing tool in aiding purification and release.

- Your animal may wish to urinate straight after or even during a healing session as the energy is processed; allow them to do so.

- Your animal may become sleepy directly after healing; allow them to rest.

- Give your animal twenty-four hours to respond to healing, as it takes this time for the energy to be assimilated throughout their body.

Whenever you are healing, go easy on yourself; allow yourself to relax and trust your intuition. Be creative; go with whatever thoughts or ideas come to you. Follow whatever makes sense to you in relation to what your pet may be feeling, and try not to be too analytical. This takes much practice, but with patience it can be achieved.

If the healing isn't working as well or as quickly as you expect, don't get disheartened. Healing works on many levels and may not necessarily work on the level which you have chosen. For instance, a physical symptom may have an emotional cause, so the healing will be absorbed greatest on the level where it's needed most.

Grounding the Healing Energy

Grounding is a vital key to a successful healing session. Grounding can be understood as securing and anchoring the healing energy that was transferred to the animal, whilst at the same time keeping any negativity out. Basically, grounding will ensure that the healing energy assimilates within the animal and stays put for a longer period of time.

Step by Step—Animal Magic Grounding Technique

After your final hand placement, move to the front of your animal client and in one steady sweep move your hands down the animal from head to tip of tail. If you are healing a horse, you must always touch the floor after a healing session; be mindful of health and safety when doing so.

Do this a total of three times.

Then flick your fingers towards the nearest door, window, or open space to discharge the energy from yourself.

Place both hands in a prayer position in the center of your chest and take three deep breaths to ground your own energy.

Step by Step—Animal Magic
Healing Disconnection Technique

After grounding your animal, step or move slightly away from your animal client.

With your hands in a prayer position at your chest area, inhale and exhale deeply a total of seven times. By doing this seven times, you are discharging any negative energy build-up from each of your chakras.

Allow each breath to resonate at your heart center, and visualize the energy moving downwards, passing through your lower chakras and resting at your root chakra, or at the base of your spine, with every exhalation.

The healing session is now complete.

Our animals bring us companionship and comfort, freedom from everyday worries, play, laughter, protection, relaxation, and peace. Help them move past anxiety, help them heal, help keep them balanced, help them feel more comfortable and relaxed, and help them enjoy their life with you. Sharing energy healing with your pet strengthens your bond together and is a fantastic way to connect with the unconditional love they share with you. You are perfectly capable of administering healing to your pet, even if you are not qualified by way of a certificate. As long as you love them unconditionally, this is enough to enable you to apply healing.

10

Crystal Spirit

As you are aware through reading this book, animals are able to connect with and communicate with most spheres of energy and energetic matter. The earth is no exception. It is thought that animals can predict changes in the earth's energy that lead up to earthquakes. I have read many accounts where bees have fled their hives and rats have left their homes in panic at such changes within the earth; it has even been reported that chickens have stopped laying eggs when there's an impending earthquake. All animals have a built-in ability to instinctively respond to escape from danger and predators to preserve their lives. They're much more finely tuned to their senses than human beings are.

The earth emits so many frequencies and vast amounts of energy that animals are instinctively attuned to it. Crystals are part of the massive energy frequency, as they form grids that span the globe, so it's little wonder that animals connect so well to the gem kingdom.

What Is a Crystal?

The word "crystal" is derived from the Greek word *krystallos*. This word means "clear ice." The word "amethyst" also derives from ancient Greece *amethystos*—meaning "unintoxicating." A crystal is a solid object whose structure is arranged in a repeating pattern.

Crystals respond in unique ways to heat, light, pressure, and sound, and can store immense amounts of information. This is also why they are used in industry, especially the quartz crystal.

How Crystals Conduct Energy

When an electrical charge or current is passed through a crystal, it is known as the piezoelectric effect. The charge changes the structure and molecules within the crystal, which change its frequency. If you take two pieces of quartz and bang them together you get sparks, although they are not going to be very bright and you may need some darkness to see them. This action stimulates piezoelectricity.

The Crystal Earth

Crystalline structure is found within the clay particles that make up the earth, the very ground that we and the animal kingdom walk upon. The total universe is based on a crystalline structure, and it is evident that all forms and all "beings" participate in this structure, no matter what their function or location in the universe. This participation is also a form of *interconnectedness*.

The Crystal Body

On a more physical level, the human body responds very well to the crystal *calcite*, as there is calcite within the pineal gland, a small endocrine gland located near the center of the brain. This area is often referred to as "the seat of the soul" or "the third eye."

A large percentage of our body is comprised of water, which is a liquid mineral that crystallizes at freezing point. Our bodies contain crystalline structures: cell salts, fatty tissue, lymph, red and white blood cells, cholesterol, etc. It is here that we can see physically, as well as psychologically, that we have strong connections with the crystal kingdom.

Quartz crystals have been growing within the earth since the earth solidified into form. It has even been suggested that quartz acts as the earth's nervous system in some way. Not all crystals we have today are as old as the earth, since crystals have been forming and reforming for millennia, but the consciousness inherent in the crystals may have access to accumulated awareness that spans the ages. Crystals can help us to remember that we are, as is everything else existing on this planet, energy, consciousness, and light.

Spirit and Matter

We can see why our ancient ancestors revered the stones of Mother Earth for use in either magical or medicinal practices, and today we can tap into their ancient wisdom and knowledge to bring about great change to ourselves and others and to the animal kingdom.

Crystals blend "spirit and matter," what I call "connecting heaven with earth." This state of being is essential for positive spiritual human development. With many light workers being "chosen" to walk in the light here on earth, spiritual essence can be transmitted into the earth's substance to affect all living creatures and make possible great planetary transformation, especially with the use of crystals. The impact of applying crystal healing to animals is felt right down to the cellular level, so the stones can even be used to help unhealthy cells gravitate towards a state of health and well-being.

Channeling crystalline energy is all about activating and integrating our light bodies and our physical forms, then blending the realities of earthly and spiritual worlds to bring healing to the animals.

Amplifying Energy

Crystals are used for healing animals as they direct, amplify, absorb, reflect, clear, transform, transmute, balance, and focus energy. You should always have a clear intention when doing crystal healing work: what result are you hoping for? Also, given that crystals can store information and energy, it is a good idea to cleanse and recharge them on a regular basis.[6] There are a variety of ways to do this, the most common being to cleanse them under running water and place them in sunlight for a number of hours, but be mindful that some crystals, like citrine, will fade when placed in sunlight and some crystals, like selenite, will disintegrate when placed in water.

Each crystal can have a number of different healing properties, and, quite often, a number of different crystals may be useful for the same specific condition. Crystals can also be applied to heal imbalances within the chakra system. It can be as simple as using a crystal the same color as the specific chakra, or as unique and complex as applying crystal matrix grids or earth alignments around an animal client for deeper, more profound healing.

Animal Healing and Geopathic Stress

Invariably, through the course of my work, I enter hundreds of houses and come into contact with acres and acres of land. As an earth acupuncturist, I am often met with displaced energies in an animal's environment, especially horses that may be sited near electricity pylons. Changes have to be made immediately in these areas too, to bring about lasting change in their health.

A woman named Melissa contacted me in September 2014 to say that her young dog, Bramble, an English Setter, had been diagnosed with bone cancer. What made this more disturbing was the fact that her

---

6   Laura Lassiter, "Crystal Connections," https://www.lauralassiter.com/blog/2016/4/25/crystal-connections.

previous three dogs had died of bone cancer too. The dogs were not of the same breed and were totally unrelated.

I instinctively knew I had to take my dowsing rods with me to see this client. Upon entering Melissa's property, I dowsed the house with my pendulum and then took out my rods. Melissa was quite surprised, as she expected that I would get straight to work with healing; however, I needed to dowse every room in the house and thankfully Melissa agreed. I detected that all but one room of her house was affected by geopathic stress. This is the theory that earth energies can be out of whack due to manmade intrusions (such as tunnels) or natural irregularities (such as geological faults) and trigger discomfort and disease in people who live in the area.

Moving outside, I saw that Melissa's dogs lived outdoors, as they were working dogs, and the rods told me that the two kennels had each been constructed over ley line intersections. Such crossed energy gives rise to the strongest effects on the physical body, which could explain the bone cancer. What transpired was that the whole of the inside of Melissa's house was affected by a swirling mass of energy. When the dogs were allowed indoors, they slept on a row of bedding along the wall touching the staircase. Melissa told me that each dog would battle over which part they were to sleep on, and Bramble, the lowest in the pecking order, always ended up sleeping at one end, the very end where I detected the highest levels of geopathic stress. The time spent with Melissa and her two dogs allowed me to place many crystal grids in quite a few areas inside her home, and three outside. I inserted quartz and copper rods at strategic places to deflect streams of energy that were having a detrimental effect on Melissa and her dogs.

Three weeks later, after a bone scan, Melissa telephoned me to say how the cellular mass had stabilized and how the dogs and Melissa felt like a major shift had taken place, as the whole feeling of their home felt light and bright.

Spare a thought as to where you place the pet beds within your home. Refrain from placing them near plug sockets and electrical items such as boilers and dishwashers, as coupled with electricity, water is also an excellent conductor of energy. Stainless steel bowls also attract electricity, so consider the dishes you allow your animals to feed from.

Finding the Earth's Core

I absolutely adore working with the earth in its purest, physical form: crystals. Not only has each gemstone taught me so much over the past twenty-odd years, but they have actually spoken to me, and also to the animals. Crystals resonate so well with all in their environment, so it's little wonder that animals are immensely aware of their healing potential. To witness an animal self-select its own crystals for healing never ceases to amaze me. Animals instinctively know the benefits that certain gems will have on their well-being.

I use crystals daily; in fact, they are as much a part of me as my right arm is. I have four cases of crystals that I take with me on location. Within each case are a vast array of gems to heal horses, dogs, cats, and smaller animals and birds; each is assigned a case.

As I grew up in Yorkshire I often found, among the ragged cliffs and landscape, little pieces of fossil and jet. However, crystals to be used for healing were something that happened quite by accident.

Stumbling on Treasure

"They're *just* pretty stones of differing colors," I remember saying at one time; that was until twenty years ago. Around five months after I suffered the stroke, I decided it was time for me to go out and face the busy world again. My very first outing was to Sheffield. I stepped out of the taxi and was met with the hustle and bustle of city life, and it almost became a little overbearing. I steadied myself and took a long, deep breath and walked towards a quieter area near the cathedral. As I walked on, my boot kicked something round in front of me and I stopped to look. It appeared to be a piece of smoked glass, pretty in appearance, so I popped it in my pocket. As I made my way around the city center another four pieces of this smoked glass appeared out of nowhere under my feet. I collected each one and met my friend Julie, who was a lecturer at the university, for lunch. When I showed her my collection of colored glass, she was amazed at all the different places around the city that they had appeared—so much so that she suggested we walk up to the university and pinpoint the places on the huge map they had in the foyer.

Earth, Air, Fire, Water, Spirit

What transpired next was truly astounding. As we pushed pins into the map, recording the places I had found the stones, we discovered that it formed a five-pointed star! The five-pointed star (or pentacle) is one of the most potent, powerful, and persistent symbols in human history. It has been important to almost every ancient culture, and in Paganism its five points symbolize earth, air, fire, water, and spirit. The pentacle is a sacred symbol, as it not only offers protection if we draw it in front of us but also is multi-faceted in its symbolism. It is present within many forms of nature and represents interconnectedness. Look within the humble apple: cut an apple in half and magically a pentacle will appear in the center. We were stunned, and when we were told that the glass was in fact smoky quartz, we could only think that something magical had occurred. I'm convinced it had!

I returned home from this memorable day, and as the internet wasn't available to me in the mid-nineties, I went to the village library and sourced the only book they had on the subject of crystals. Amazed with my discovery, I decided to research smoky quartz. This wasn't an easy task twenty-odd years ago, as crystals weren't as popular as they are today. Books on the subject were few and far between, except for books that took on a more scientific slant. I was thankful to find the one and only book about crystals in my local library. The little book told me all I needed to know and unearthed such mystery behind my smoky quartz treasures.

My eyes skipped from paragraph to paragraph. I discovered that smoky quartz is all about removing negativity, often through crisis, and how it is a grounding and centering stone. As I read further, I learned that smoky quartz is a root chakra stone, enhancing survival instincts. Another message, as I was determined to survive that stroke! What a magical stone to have found its way into my life, and at a time I needed its wisdom the most! Furthermore, on an emotional level, smoky quartz is excellent for elevating moods, overcoming negative emotions, relieving depression, stress, fear, jealousy, anger, etc.

I was perplexed for many weeks, wondering how and why these magical stone pieces had lain upon the floor ready for me to find on that particular day. Twenty-plus years on, I still haven't found the answer! This initial connection to smoky quartz led me to seek out further stones and crystals and also to further my knowledge of them. By tapping into the wisdom of the crystal world, I wanted to learn of the possibility of animals connecting with their energy too. This was the very start of my crystal journey.

Shamanic Connection

Through a friend of a friend (as is often the case), I was given the contact details of a man named Boo. Boo had been raised in an Aborigine family; his father was a shaman (similar to a Druid high priest) who worked closely with the earth. Aborigines believe some of their ancestors metamorphosed into nature (as in rock formations or rivers), where they remain spiritually alive, so it's not difficult to understand how these indigenous tribespeople have a natural affinity with the crystal world.

To illustrate the point above, Boo spoke to his long-deceased father through a piece of rock he carried with him at all times. Boo's father connected deeply with the animal kingdom when he was alive and spoke of how, at the age of eight, he had his life totem animal or spirit animal "sung" into him and was blessed with the powers of heron. This totem bird served to protect him and nourish his spirit, and the heron totem remained within the man until death.

With the blessing of his father rock, Boo found himself on a personal pilgrimage around Britain, the first time that he had ventured from the Australian outback. Through his visions, meditations, and inward journeys, Boo had been "called" by his soul to seek the energy of the stone circles, cairns, chambers, and other sacred sites across the British Isles.

I made contact with Boo whilst he was traveling the West Penwith area of Cornwall. This magical county of the UK is steeped in legend, myth, and folklore and is home to many ancient and sacred sites, from holy wells to stone circles.

I needed to learn more about the crystal kingdom, and after I had connected with Boo I knew he was the person to teach me. Surprisingly, Boo was much older than I anticipated: seventy-seven. We agreed to meet the following week in Derbyshire at a small sacred stone circle called Doll Tor that is little known about; I couldn't wait.

The Original Aboriginal Shaman

My friend and I made our way to Stanton in the Peak, a small village on the outskirts of the world-famous pudding town of Bakewell. I felt very lucky to have the rolling hills of the Derbyshire Peaks on my doorstep, and the numerous sacred circles, marker stones, and ancient trackways in this beautiful county.

I pulled the car over and took out a picnic blanket from the boot, and we made our way up the narrow track to the ancient settlement. As we were taking in the scenery of the surrounding moorland we heard the most amazing vocal sounds and piped music coming from up ahead. We reached our destination of the tiny sacred circle and it was there we were met with the most incredible and prodigious sight. Spread out on a huge handwoven, silk-embroidered, cream-colored cloth was a vast array of crystals, and sitting within the center was Boo. The etheric sounds of pipe and chant that Boo was creating merged beautifully with the crystals and soothed our ears as we spread out our picnic blankets upon the warm, damp earth beside him. It was officially the end of British summertime, but for me it felt like a new chapter in my new life had just begun.

Crystal Application

When applying crystals for healing with animals, there are a number of techniques you can adapt to suit each species; here is just a sample:

- **Channeled healing:** A relevant crystal is held in the hands of the healer, and the healing energy is channeled through the crystal.

- **Direct healing:** The crystal is placed touching the fur, feathers, or scales of an animal, and the healer allows the crystal to do the healing.

- **Crystal grids:** A variety of crystals are placed in a responding grid around the animal's body (not suitable for horses or larger animals in confined spaces, due to health and safety issues).

- **Constant healing:** Crystals are placed in a collar, saddle, or under the bed of an animal to allow for constant healing.

Neddy—The Self-Selector

Neddy was a three-year-old mixed terrier breed. He had become infirm at just two years old after developing a muscular condition shortly after his annual vaccination. Justine, his owner, was a very spiritual woman and wanted to give holistic treatment a try, rather than just administering long-term medication to her beloved dog.

Neddy greeted me at the door like I was a long-lost friend, chirping and turning slowly round in circles. He shared his home with another companion, Tutu, a Westie. It became apparent that even though Neddy had undergone numerous veterinary investigations, his exact medical diagnosis had proven inconclusive.

Bearing in mind the information Justine had given me, I selected around fifteen crystals from my case and placed them on my cloth upon the wooden floor. I took out my pendulum, as I had intended to dowse over each crystal, which would enable me to select the most beneficial ones for Neddy: to aid his mobility, reduce pain, and stimulate his energy return. However, I'd only just managed to take out my pendulum from its pouch when Neddy slowly came over to me, sniffed each crystal in turn, licked five of them, and lay down with his head resting over my lap as if to say, "Okay, let's get started." Justine laughed as I remarked how Neddy seemed to be a no-nonsense sort of chap!

Neddy enjoyed a total of five crystal therapy sessions; each time, he self-selected the crystals he needed, in his own unique way. As I arrived to give Neddy his fifth and final treatment, Justine met me at the door armed with a series of photographs. In each one Neddy was jumping on logs, running through the autumn leaves, and leaping over woodland logs with his sister, Tutu!

At the time of writing this book I am still in touch with Justine, who keeps me updated on all Neddy's adventures!

Animal Magic Crystal Therapy

Applying crystal therapy with animals, and seeing the incredible and almost miraculous results, led me to develop my practitioner course for this modality. Because of the unique nature of the training, it took me four years. It is now the only Animal Crystal Therapy distance-learning course offering a professional diploma qualification in the UK.

A typical healing session generally involves the animal lying down while crystals are placed on or near to the chakras and also around the body in various matrix layouts. This method is more effective for healing cats and dogs. Unfortunately, the nature of the horse does not lend itself to such a treatment, so we use techniques that involve either holding the crystals over the horse's body or moving the crystals throughout the aura.

If you wish to give healing with crystals a try with your own animals, below are my favorite eight starter stones, along with the key ailments they can help.

Carnelian

- Relieves bowel problems
- Aids in recovery from operations
- Strengthens the human-animal bond
- Good for pack leader problems/boisterous animals
- Helps with spinal issues
- Good for stomach and digestive issues

Green Aventurine

- For overall health balancing
- For endurance or agility
- Grounds negative or excessive energies
- Relieves anxiety
- Calms the nervous system
- For hyperactivity

Blue Calcite

- Helps with sleep issues
- Aids in arthritis

- Good for respiratory issues
- Helps repair muscular tissues
- Settles animals during travel
- Assists with mobility

Amethyst

- For nervousness and shyness
- For thyroid problems
- For blood disorders
- For animals that have separation anxiety
- To calm animals always on the go
- For animals that dominate others/animals

Clear Quartz

- For animals who have come from rescue centers
- For over-stimulated minds
- For ear problems and deafness
- For blindness
- For epilepsy and neurological issues
- For mouth and teeth problems
- To help animals pass to the Rainbow Bridge

Ajoite

- Brings the highest vibrational energies for healing—
  separates the physical body of the healer from the process
  and utilizes spiritual energy only

- Encourages animals to become guides on earth for other animals
- Removes negative attachments that hinder the physical body's healing
- Enables the animal to connect any past life with that of their human

Sunstone

- Stimulates vitality, especially post-operative
- Brings healing to the lower chakras
- Helps relieve stress stimulated by other animals within the environment
- Promotes energy when competing
- Filters toxins from the environment, e.g., geopathic stress
- Increases the healing potential of other crystals in grids

Flint

- Enhances the ability for animals to communicate their feelings to humans
- Promotes self-respect
- Helps create a "clean start" after a period of abuse
- Helps the animal communicator contact energy from the animal's past lives
- Enables boundaries to stay in place
- Heals animals who've suffered trauma from giving birth

Crystal Considerations

When giving crystal therapy to an animal, it is important to consider the following, especially if you or your animals are new to the healing energy of crystals:

- Be prepared for your animals to be inquisitive around the crystals; you may have to split the healing session into small chunks.

- Will you use a combination of crystal applications for mind, body, and spirit, or will you work on just one level, or just over a physical area of the body?

- Will you be applying the crystals directly upon your animal or placing them around the animal? If placing crystals upon them, do your own research, as some crystals are toxic.

- Consider the size of crystal you are using in relation to your animal. Crystals that are very small can easily be swallowed.

- Be prepared for nervousness! Animals are very sensitive creatures so there may be some crystals' energy they readily accept and others they do not. Never force an animal to be near a crystal.

- Will you allow the animal to self-select crystals? This can be done by simply holding a crystal in each palm and observing the animal's interest in them.

- Ensure your crystals have been washed and cleansed, and never use the same crystal with another animal without cleansing it first.

Step by Step—Getting Animals
Accustomed to Crystal Energy

Find a place where you will not be disturbed, preferably when your animal has eaten a meal.

Sit (if you're working with a companion animal) or stand (if you're working with a horse) beside your animal and take three deep breaths.

Select your cleansed crystal and allow your animal to look at it, and maybe sniff it.

If the animal stays within the presence of the crystal, then you may go ahead with the session. If your animal walks away, then this may not be the time to apply crystal healing, or you may wish to try again with a different crystal.

Hold the crystal in your closed palm, close your eyes, and allow yourself to feel its resonance. Notice the energy it's emitting within your palm. Be aware of how it makes you feel. To give an effective crystal healing treatment, *you* also need to be attuned to the energy of the stone you are using.

Open your eyes and take a breath in and out, and open your palm, allowing the energy of the crystal to flow outwards towards your animal.

You may wish to hold the crystal over a specific area of the animal's body, by making contact with your animal with light pressure.

Just allow the energy to flow, observing your animal as you do so. You will instinctively know if the crystal energy is a pleasant experience for your pet.

After the session, close your palm and place your other hand over it. This grounds the energy of the crystal.

Put the crystal in a safe place and stroke your animal from head to tail three times; this grounds the energy of the animal.

Place your hands together at your heart center and take in three deep, releasing breaths; this grounds your own energy.

Direct Healing with Quartz

If your animal has a weakness in a particular area, you can use two single-terminated quartz crystals (in other words, crystals that have a single pointed end) rather than only using one crystal. Utilizing crystals in this way can improve energy flow within a blocked area of the body. This simple crystal healing technique can be implemented at any part of the body, but in my experience it is particularly suitable for treating leg problems such as tissue tears, ruptured muscle, or trapped nerves.

Method

Hold a single-terminated quartz crystal on each side of the damaged area. You need the points facing the animal's leg, so the crystals should be facing towards each other.

Hold the points in position for ten to fifteen minutes.

Three treatments are advisable for this method, usually once a day for three consecutive days.

Obviously, crystal healing should be used only after you have a diagnosis from your vet. Crystals can be used as a supplementary healing aid to your vet's recommendations, but should not be considered a substitute for orthodox care.

Having crystals throughout our living environment is a fantastic way for animals to experience all that crystal energy can offer, passively. Just as plants and animals in the wild benefit from areas where the crystals lie naturally, our pets will also gain from crystals we intentionally place around our home.

11
Reiki

As a professional animal healer, and, unusually, one with a scientific background, I understand that holistic healing shouldn't work, at least by all medical and scientific laws. But it does, and my recovery from the stroke shows that I am living proof of that. Even the most skeptical amongst us cannot deny that great miracles have been performed throughout history within the realm of healing.

For conventional doctors, natural healing is a very misunderstood concept. Most medical professionals have spent numerous years in training, learning all about the physical body and its functions, leaving little room for the more energetic roles. However, over the past twenty years of my work as a healer, things have undergone great change, especially in relation to complementary medicine for animals.

I have been lucky to teach people from all walks of life, including medical professionals and general practitioners. One such student who was learning animal communication was a GP from Cambridge. This particular gentleman was of Hindu faith and expressed his comfort in class at being among like-minded souls, people who were *believers* in the universal power of healing; people just like him. He attended my

Soul Speak Animal Communication course to help him become more in tune with his tortoiseshell cat, who was an absolute sweetie. After learning a few basic techniques, he was amazed at the positive responses he received as he soon became in direct communication with his cat back home. Furthermore, when I started teaching about the power of the pendulum in animal communication, he began trying to figure out how he could incorporate the pendulum into his general practice, as he was astounded at the results during the practical demonstrations!

Many people who walk the spiritual path are demystifying healing, which is making it more accessible and acceptable for all people and their animals. Healing is as old as humankind; its unrivaled universal energy wasn't a misunderstood phenomenon for our ancestors, but a power source that was used daily. The hands-on healing approach was all the ancients had available to them, along with their beliefs that the Great Spirit would assist them back to full health. Their beliefs also incorporated the premise that any physical illness was the creation of an unhealthy soul or spirit, and many holistic healers still believe in this concept today.

Modern Medicine

When modern medicine treats humans on a purely physical level, it restricts healing in other areas of the *being*. Holistic healing, of course, nourishes the soul, which promotes the healing of spirit, which in turn can stimulate the self-healing mechanism of the physical body. All forms of natural healing are increasing in popularity at a very great rate, and I believe this is because medical science isn't adequately meeting the needs or supporting the beliefs of people and their animals; people may require a different type of medicine, one without side effects and that doesn't just treat the symptoms.

Persecution for Believing

Throughout history, healers have been persecuted for practicing their beliefs in natural medicine. As well as having their healing powers disbelieved, they were accused of being witches, and it was believed that their healing powers made them associates of the devil. Thankfully times have changed, though we still have many people who doubt the positive changes that healing can bring. Skeptics are my best form of advertising, however, because once they have seen what healing can do, they come to understand and accept it, and then cannot wait to tell everyone about the "miracle."

Rebirth through Reiki

When I was resting on the sofa one day recovering from the stroke, my cat Sophie began to paw the edge of a book about Reiki. I pulled the book from the bottom of the pile and, as I thumbed through it, it was as though I was making a connection with a long-lost friend. As I read further, the words on every page resonated with me. I knew this was going to be a breakthrough, and the very opportunity I was seeking to heal myself.

The Universal Life Force

"Reiki" refers to the vibrational, universal life force energy that is harnessed and channeled through the hands of the Reiki healer into the recipient. The Japanese word *Rei* is translated as "essence" or "soul," and *Ki* is "energy." I feel that Reiki is an uplifting gift that connects us to our true essence. Through it, the higher self can connect to universal energy. The research I did helped me to understand how we are all connected—how we are all made of molecules vibrating at different rates—and it spoke the knowledge of our ancestors. Reiki is an energy that empowers every living thing.

Reiki Empowerment

Humankind has been aware of the presence of life force energy for thousands of years. We carry it in and around our bodies, even though we are often not aware of it. Eastern traditions have strived to channel and apply it in a variety of disciplines—such as Reiki, Tai Chi, Feng Shui, meditation, yoga, and acupuncture—which focus on controlling and enhancing the flow of this energy. The Reiki energy itself is considered to have an "omniscient wisdom" that anyone, no matter what faith or religion, is capable of tapping into.

Unlike spiritual healing, Reiki relies on no particular faith or belief system, although to be able to channel Reiki energy one needs to receive an attunement via a Reiki Master. More often than not, you will be guided to this master at the right time, when you are ready to accept what the study of Reiki has to offer. As I myself discovered, it is almost as if Reiki itself takes the active step of finding you.[7]

Introducing Reiki

My introduction to Reiki was in 1995. Without the internet, I had the arduous task of finding a Reiki Master who could offer me healing and maybe attune me to Reiki to help aid my further recovery from the stroke. My quest led me twenty miles or so to the Peak District, where I stumbled upon a wonderful Reiki Master, a woman named Janet, quite by accident. This enlightened soul enabled me to experience the Reiki energy that I had until then only read about.

Reiki healing activated my own personal Ki and accelerated my healing greatly, aiding in my full recovery without the need of drugs; even the medical professionals were amazed at the hastened improvement of my physical and mental health. Through Reiki I could rationalize the stroke, and I began to realize that my "pre-stroke" life had

---

7   Adele Malone and Gary Malone, *The Essence of Reiki: Usui Reiki Levels 1, 2, 3,* 2018.

become fragmented and hollow. I understood that my body had reacted to this emotional fragmentation with physical interference, stopping me in my tracks and provoking me to take action to address all the imbalances in my life. The human body is a wise teacher, and pursuing its wisdom through Reiki allowed me to grow to new heights of understanding. My life began to flow freely and with ease.

Attuning to Life

I am forever grateful that Mikao Usui re-founded the healing practice of Reiki in the early 1900s and that it was brought to the Western world by Hawayo Takata. There are many different theories about how Reiki was discovered by Usui, but the fact of the matter is that his legacy has been this amazing system of energy work that has healed thousands of humans and animals over the last decade.

My three years of going from Reiki level one up to Reiki Master Teacher saw me healing not only myself but many others too. I became sensitive to my own needs and was compelled to help others change their lives as well. My Reiki healing attunements were taken in sacred spaces in Derbyshire, England, upon the ancient land and amidst the stone circles of our ancestors. The series of attunements, over three years, to this amazing energy gave me the strength and courage to shift my perspective from external needs to my own internal requirements.

Because Reiki is holistic, it had a major impact on my body, my mind, and my spirit, giving me the ability to heal myself and recognize what I needed to do to amplify my own recovery. For me, it released blocked emotional and physical elements that had led me to my suffering the stroke, things I had pushed to the back of my mind yet my body insisted on holding on to.

For me, Reiki brought pure unconditional love, along with learning; it also brought joy and enlightenment, and I embraced it.

The Way of Reiki

To enable the user of Reiki to be enhanced by its energy, Usui developed a set of principles for the healer to follow that help you connect to the energy of Reiki at all times, even when not applying healing. Adopting these precepts adds balance and substance to life. However, it is important to realize that we are not *expected* to live every moment of our lives within the framework of these ideals. As humans we are all imperfect, and that is why each of the principles begins with "Just for today." You can, without pressure or stress, work on improving yourself daily. If you make a mistake today, you can always begin again tomorrow. The more you work with the principles, the more you will condition yourself to adopt them as a way of life, just as I do.

The Five Reiki Principles by Mikao Usui will have different meanings for each individual. Meditation is one way to help to unlock your personal understandings of each one.

The Five Reiki Principles

1. Just for today I will not worry

2. Just for today I will not be angry

3. Just for today I will do my work honestly

4. Just for today I will give thanks for my many blessings

5. Just for today I will be kind to my neighbor and every living thing

Just for Today I Will Not Worry

Stress and worry are the primary reasons for the build-up of tension in the body. Anxiety can block the root chakra and throw your body, mind, and spirit out of balance. But we are not helpless; we have a choice in how to respond to life's difficulties. If we react in a knee-jerk, negative way, we are in effect allowing damage to the mind, body, and spirit. Rather, take a deep breath and try to look at the problem as an opportunity to learn, like I did with the stroke. Choosing to respond positively will enable you to live a richer, more joyful life.

Just for Today I Will Not Be Angry

Anger can cause stomach and intestinal problems and is generally a toxic emotion. To release yourself from anger, the first thing to understand is what causes it. Once the triggers are identified, you can take your power back by finding new ways to approach situations, turning what could be a negative experience into a positive. Again, this involves making a choice and not let this destructive emotion drain your energy. Once you take this step, other things in your life will improve.

Just for Today I Will Do My Work Honestly

Our understanding of honesty and dishonesty can run the gamut from little white lies to destructive deception. While an obvious example of not being honest would be to steal someone else's property, it's also important to realize that not all forms of stealing involve other people; sometimes we steal from ourselves, which is in effect being dishonest with ourselves. For example, don't steal valuable time from yourself by wasting it on things that don't matter, such as playing games on electronic devices. And don't steal from yourself by not pursuing your talents and passions in this life.

Just for Today I Will Give Thanks For My Many Blessings

It has been said that needs and wants are different, and that while we may not get the latter, we will get the former. I never look on the traumatic event of the stroke as something that I didn't need. Quite the opposite—it was *exactly* what I needed, as it brought to me understanding, learning, and inner knowledge that set me on the inner path and brought me to where I am today: happy. If, rather than complaining about the difficulties we face, we make a conscious effort to understand that each challenge is a chance to grow and blossom, it will move us toward spiritual enlightenment. Take a moment to smell the roses and appreciate the blessings in your life: your animal friends, for one!

Just for Today I Will Be Kind to My Neighbor and Every Living Thing

I'm sure we've all heard the offhand popular saying, "What goes around, comes around." But there is a profound truth to this. The energy you send out, whether positive—kindness, love—or negative—anger, resentment—will in some way boomerang back to you. Accepting this idea can help us to live a more peaceful and positive life, in that we can help to shape our own experiences through our actions.[8]

The Path to Reiki

I followed my path to Reiki in my quest for healing. I desired to make my own decisions about my well-being without relying on prescription medicine or orthodox treatment. Others might come to Reiki simply in search of proactive, positive change in their life, or even on the recommendation of a friend. Perhaps they are skeptics, or skeptical, but are willing to try something new to combat a feeling of drifting or emptiness. When I found Reiki, it helped me put all the pieces of my fragmented life back together in a brand-new order.

The secret to getting the most from Reiki is to be open to its energy. The key, as longtime practitioners and teachers know, to becoming a Reiki enthusiast is to be receptive to its energy and "allow the joy of Reiki to envelop you ... Trust in the omniscient wisdom of Reiki."[9] I did, and I have never looked back. Let yourself realize that you are following this path because you should be. Your intuition is a wonderful guide as you search for what direction you should go.

---

8   Descriptions of the five principles based on *The Essence of Reiki* by Adele and Gary Malone.

9   Malone, *The Essence of Reiki.*

The Reiki Ceremony or Attunement

Reiki is very different than other healing modalities. It progresses in stages, and the first step is to undertake the first degree initiation ceremony. (This level enables you to perform healing on family and friends; higher levels enable you to work professionally.) The level one ceremony consists firstly in learning the Reiki modality; the attunement is given at the end of the training. This process also allows the student to feel, sense, and experience the Reiki energy firsthand.

When I was out in Derbyshire, surrounded by ancient standing stones, my experience of level one attunement was a deeply personal one. The ancient landmark of Doll Tor, hidden away in a copse of native British trees, had many stories to tell about the ancient people who sat in the very same spot as I. The cold earth anchored my energy into the ground and I felt alive; my whole body had never felt so connected and so conscious. The whole Reiki process, which took over three years, was almost like a rite of passage, facilitating a total connection to myself, my needs, my own inner healing, and life itself.

Reiki Symbols

Another way in which Reiki is unlike any other healing system is in the use of its symbols. During a typical Reiki attunement process, the Master uses ancient Reiki symbols and mantras (holy words that activate and direct certain energies) to connect the student to the universal life force of Reiki. You will never lose this energy after you have been connected to it!

Within the traditional Usui system of Reiki, there are four sacred symbols from ancient Sanskrit text. The symbols make this system of healing unique, as healing energy is channeled through them, unlike in other applications of healing where energy is channeled simply through the laying-on of hands. The passing of symbols from Reiki Master to student usually involves the symbols being drawn by a finger (or visualized in the mind's eye) by the Reiki Master and placed in specific areas of the energy field of the student's body, including the crown chakra, third eye, and palms of the hands. The Reiki Master also blows the symbols by breath and often taps the symbols physically upon the initiate's palms. Because the Reiki symbols are unique and a physical concept that can be visualized during a healing session, they strengthen the connection to Reiki as an energy, bringing about a more profound healing session. As the keys that unlock the flow of Reiki and enhance and amplify the Reiki energy, the symbols help the Reiki practitioner connect more effectively to the universal life force.

During my Reiki One attunement, the birds were singing loudly and I saw my totem bird, a jay, flit between the branches of an ancient oak tree, along with chaffinches and long-tailed tits. It was obvious that all my senses were awakening. The bird song seemed to be greatly enhanced and became almost hypnotic. I could hear each blade of grass move and sway in the gentle breeze, and when I opened my eyes after the ceremony, it was as if I was seeing nature for the very first time. The leaves of the overhanging boughs seemed to be colored with iridescent green foliage, a green I had failed to see before this moment. The whole experience for me was an awakening of mind, body, and spirit.

The traditional Reiki symbol meaning:

- **Cho Ku Rei:** This is the power symbol.

- **Sei Hi Ki:** This is mental and emotional symbol.

- **Hon Sha Ze Sho Nen:** This is the distant healing symbol.

- **Dai Ko Myo:** This is used by Reiki Masters to empower the other symbols and when attuning others.

Reiki Guides

An interesting aspect of Reiki is the guides that accompany you during the journey. Do not be surprised if ancestors, elemental beings, earth spirits, angels, and spirit guides sense your activity and come to assist you. The main role of these beings is to provide important healing information, which is especially beneficially if you are giving Reiki to clients. For example, the guides may indicate a spot on the body that would most benefit from Reiki healing, or convey insight about why an area is out of balance or in a state of "dis-ease." They can even help you come up with ideas, or recommendations for your client, on how to address the energetic imbalances that have been identified. Being in touch with the guides can make a big difference in the level of healing you are able to provide.[10]

The Need for Attunement

The Reiki attunement opens the crown chakra, the heart chakra, and the chakras located within the palms. Along with the ancient Reiki symbols placed into your energy field during the attunement process, the Reiki Master opens the chakras through your crown, activating each one to enable the Reiki energy to flow within you.

The Self-Cleansing Process

After the first attunement, Reiki energy starts to flow through the hands whenever you become aware of it. A twenty-one day cleansing, transformation, and detoxification cycle also begins. This cleansing influences the whole chakra system, beginning with the root chakra and finalizing at the crown, each one taking approximately three days; hence the period of twenty one days.

My Personal Cleansing Release

I wasn't aware, after my attunement, of any chakra transformation allowing a release from my own body. However, I was aware that certain

---

10   Melanie Jacobs, "Reiki and the Chakras: a Gateway for Opening Spiritual Gifts," https://iarp.org/reiki-and-the-chakras-gateway-for-opening -spiritual-gifts/.

areas of my life and my emotional body needed to be readjusted, rebalanced, and realigned with each other. My personal transformation happened on day twelve of the twenty-one day cleansing period. Until day twelve I'd felt extremely energized; I felt happy, healthy, and well. In fact, you could say that I became positive that I would pass through this transformation period "unwounded."

How wrong I was! I was shopping in Sainsbury's and all was well, until I pushed my trolley down the dairy aisle. Instantly I became very emotional. I took out a tissue from my bag and dabbed at my nose; I started to sniff and then my eyes started to run. I knew this was something more than a chill from the fridge cabinets and became very embarrassed as I clung on to my trolley. Then my legs gave way, and a kind lady alerted a member of the staff, who brought over a security guard. Initially they thought that I'd had my bag stolen. I was in a heap on the floor and I could not stop crying; my whole body was shaking.

Throughout the whole incident, memories from my childhood, my teens, and my adulthood were replaying in my mind. I couldn't understand what was happening to me. Obscure thoughts were running through my head, and most of them involved negative experiences. As I look back I now understand that this was my own personal "crisis" or cleansing. I needed to go through it to be cleansed and come out the other side.

I received my second degree in Reiki one year later, on the magical date of Midsummer. As our small group gathered in the forest clearing, the sun shone through the branches of a majestic oak tree, preparing us for a new way of being.

The Three Degrees of Reiki

It was the early 1990s when I became attuned to the first degree of Reiki. Back then, the student had to wait one year before embarking on the remaining journey. This was to allow the energy to develop and manifest within the healer.

After my Reiki Two attunement, a further two years had to pass before I could take the mastership level, with another six months before I could apply to become a Master Teacher. I practiced, practiced, and practiced! Each student who attended Reiki training at that time had to give over a hundred Reiki treatments before even being considered to do Master training.

I've been a Master Teacher for over twenty years now. My lineage line is pure and I'm lucky enough to be just eleventh on the lineage tree from the founder of this unique energy: Mikao Usui.

The Reiki levels are:

- **Shoden is Reiki One:** Reiki for yourself and family and friends. No symbols are given within your training manual.

- **Okuden is Reiki Two:** This enables you to work professionally. Three symbols are given with training.

- **Shinpiden is Reiki Mastership:** One final symbol is given to you to complete the other three symbols, which heightens your healing ability.

- **Reiki Master Teacher:** This enables you to attune others in the tradition of Reiki.

Reiki One

After receiving your first degree attunement from a Reiki Master, you are prepared to work with the universal life force. (But as in any profession, keep in mind that it is important to master the fundamentals before progressing to the next level.) Your intuition with grow as you work with the Reiki energy, and your own vibration will rise. In terms of your daily life, you will find yourself experiencing a pleasing sense of consistency.

Reiki Two

There are three symbols that are taught to students during the second degree training. As with your connection to the life force energy, after you have been attuned to the symbols you will be connected to them for life, whether at a conscious or subconscious level. And, even if you are not trying to use the symbols while doing Reiki healing, they will flow through you. To what extent you want to employ the symbols in your practice is up to you, and something you will get a better sense of as your understanding of Reiki grows.

Reiki Master Training

There is an additional symbol to conclude Reiki training, which completes the whole system of Reiki.

Symbol Empowerment

Once you have reached Reiki Two and assimilated the first three symbols, their healing powers increases. Without actually undergoing the second degree attunement, the symbols will not work. Regardless, rest assured that the Reiki symbols, like Reiki energy, can never cause any harm! Their only power is for the good.[11]

Reiki in Practice

Because Reiki works on all levels of the mind, body, and spirit, the releasing process can be quite powerful emotionally, as well as tiring. The energy needs to address the blocks, wounds, and "baggage" that your body has spent a lifetime accumulating. But rest assured that the wisdom of Reiki will do whatever is necessary to free you from those obstacles that stand in the way of you living your best life.[12]

---

11   Descriptions of Reiki levels based on *The Essence of Reiki* by Adele and Gary Malone.

12   *Reiki 1 Manual: A Complete Guide to the First Degree Usui Method of Natural Healing*, 2014.

To Give Reiki is to Receive Reiki

One of the major differences between Reiki and other forms of healing is that Reiki is never sent; it is *channeled* through the symbols into the recipient. Because of this, the Reiki practitioner will never feel drained or take on the condition, illness, or ailment of the recipient. On the contrary, the practitioner is also receiving a treatment as the Reiki energy flows through them.

Self-Healing with Reiki

Since Reiki teaches the importance of self-healing, it is necessarily a starting point for insight into yourself. Additionally, it provides you with the ability for self-protection and personal transformation in a multitude of ways. Of course, during and after your Reiki work, you will still encounter the same daily difficulties as before; you may have changed, but life didn't! Yet with your connection to Reiki energy, you will have the tools and understanding to surmount the challenges that come your way. Even if your Reiki healing practice is a purely personal one, not something you use to heal others, you will experience a profound new sense of balance and wisdom.[13]

Animals and Reiki

Treating animals with Reiki is very different from healing with the Animal Magic healing system. While in Animal Magic we heal with energy bands, in Reiki there are set hand positions, held for a period of time before moving on to another position. All animals respond very well to Reiki, and because there are symbols to use within the system, you are able to focus the energy on specific goals. For example, there is a symbol specifically for emotional healing, whilst another is for applying healing from a distance. Reiki is a wonderful healing energy to use with small animals like mice, hamsters, guinea pigs, etc., as you can just cup your

13   Malone, *The Essence of Reiki.*

hands gently around their bodies, without pressure. You are also able to treat animals within cages (such as birds and reptiles) with Reiki, as it's a soft and passive energy that most animals enjoy being part of.

If you are interested in exploring Reiki to heal your own pets, the first step would be to get a Reiki One attunement. If you wish to work with Reiki for animals on the professional level, however, be sure to research the licensing requirements in your country. In the UK, it is mandatory that the healer be trained in six modules; there are currently practitioners who find themselves in court for practicing Reiki with animals when not adequately trained to do so.

Gratitude

Reiki led me onto the path I walk today; the path of love and healing, and for this I will be eternally grateful. Thank you, Reiki.

12

The Pendulum

Dowsing is a practice that is probably as old as mankind itself. It has been passed down the generations for all manner of things, including being used to detect unexploded bombs, by oil companies to detect underground fuel sources, by practitioners to locate cures for illnesses, by psychics who wish to divine future events, by construction companies to check whether foundations are in place on which to create building developments, and by individuals to establish what foods will be of benefit to us.

I have personally been thrown many an inquiring look in the supermarket or grocery store as I dowse over the fruit and herbal tea section to determine the one I need at that time. Working with a pendulum in relation to personal health matters or healing animals does take an amount of practice to become proficient at, but it provides dividends when giving you the answers to your many questions.

The Pineal Gland

It is thought that dowsers use the pineal gland when using a pendulum. The pineal gland is a pea-shaped mass behind the brain, and some studies believe that this is actually the third eye. Oddly, the pineal gland has all of the components needed for a functioning eye. There may be a small possibility that when our ancients spoke of a "third eye" they knew what they were talking about. The pineal gland is also thought to secrete a chemical known as DMT, which has been nicknamed "the spirit molecule." DMT is believed to be released whilst we dream, throughout spiritual and mystical experiences, during meditation, and in the time before death.

While there isn't any proof that the pineal gland is a spiritual eye seeing into other dimensions, it is fascinating that it has the biological potential to be an actual eye. When one looks inwards, as with dowsing and other forms of mind stillness and spiritual awareness, the pineal gland becomes active; hence, this gland plays an effective part in any dowsing work you undertake.

Our Subconscious Mind

The subconscious mind is a powerhouse of all our thoughts and experiences. It stores everything, even the things we are unaware of or think we don't notice. The subconscious, as well as taking over during spiritual experiences, plays an integral part in our waking state too; for instance, when driving a car. At one stage whilst learning to drive, one couldn't have ever thought that they would have been able to hold a conversation whilst driving; yet a year or less on the road and we're letting our subconscious mind drive the car automatically, changing gears, making observations, etc., whilst our conscious mind is chatting away to passengers.

Dowsing and Animal Healing

For me, the pendulum plays an integral part in the majority of my healing work, but especially when I'm working with animals. Below are some of the key areas where using a pendulum is vital:

- To determine if an animal wants to be part of the healing process

- To detect auric impurities

- To select the most appropriate method of healing for a specific animal: for example, crystal therapy, Reiki, or flower/plant essences

- To provide information on which body area to focus on: for example, physical, emotional, etc.

- To determine the cause of any allergies

- To check whether the overall healing treatment has been successful

Pendulum Types

Dowsing pendulums can be purchased, or can be made from most things you may have lying around your house. A key on a piece of string, a ring dangling from a length of chain, a bead on a piece of ribbon; all these are good dowsing tools to start with. There are a wide range of pendulums available in all manner of shapes, sizes, and materials. My personal favorites are crystal pendulums. I have a particular favorite, a snow quartz pendulum that has been with me for my animal healing work for over ten years now. Snow quartz is also known as milky quartz. It is a gentle, calming stone and enhances meditation by allowing the user to link to deep inner wisdom; you can see why this never fails to support me in my work with animals.

The Moving Pendulum

The pendulum works individually for each user. This means that the pendulum will indicate yes/no answers differently depending on the handler. For me and most people, pendulums will always rotate clockwise for an affirmative answer and spin counterclockwise to indicate "no." If the pendulum moves from a top to bottom motion, this tells me the answers to questions I am asking in relation to specific health concerns for the animal I am working with. If my pendulum moves from left to right, it indicates that I need to investigate the question further. I have found through teaching pendulum methods that for left-handed people the pendulum will usually work in a totally opposite way than for right handed people. So the counterclockwise rotation will probably indicate an affirmative answer. Give it a go and see what you get! The pendulum really does open up a whole new avenue in healing.

Holding the Pendulum
Pinch your pendulum between your forefinger and thumb.

If you find it more comfortable, you may wish to hold the chain over your middle finger between the joints and steady it with your thumb.

Another option is to hold it between forefinger and middle finger, and allow the chain to rest over your thumb to steady the pendulum for maximum control.

Approaches in Questioning the Pendulum
When you start to use a pendulum, you need to be aware that direct questions are almost always the best form of probing. Don't try and use a whole sentence to ask the pendulum one thing. Use direct questioning and avoid joining words. You need to be precise when making requests. If your question isn't specific, your answer will be vague.

Connecting with Your Pendulum
I always start by developing an initial bond with my pendulum. This is a simple exercise in which I ask the pendulum a question that I already know the answer to. So for instance, "In this lifetime, is my name Niki?" The pendulum will then answer "yes" and start to spin clockwise. I then know that the pendulum is willing to work with me at that point in time.

Step by Step—Attuning the Pendulum

Your pendulum will work for you if you are working without ego and for the highest good of the animal. To establish if an animal wishes to be given healing, follow these steps:

Ensure that you have cleansed your pendulum (e.g., by running it under tepid water and not having used it with another animal since cleansing).

Connect with it yourself before placing it within the animal's energy field.

Enable the animal to connect with the pendulum too by allowing him or her to sniff it.

Ask your pendulum a question that you know the answer to; this will establish if it's going to be appropriate to use it at that time, during your particular healing session.

Always start by pendulum dowsing at the side of the animal's body near the head area, and work towards the tail; be aware that if you are dowsing over a cat they may think the pendulum chain is another toy to play with!

Holding your arm and hand as still as possible, ask your intended question and wait a few moments for the response. For example, "Does Tilly want healing today?"

Accept the answer.

When Pendulums Won't Work

In 2002 I discovered the crystal moss agate. How excited was I to learn that moss agate is also known as the Druid Stone. I made it my mission to undertake a search for a piece of this, as I felt sure it was going to serve me well and connect deeply with me; after all, I was a Druid!

After searching for a few months I came across a moss agate dowsing pendulum in a New Age shop in Derbyshire. Thankful that my search was over, I paid for the pendulum and popped it in my handbag. As soon as I arrived home, I looked for it in my bag but it was nowhere to be found. I checked my coat pocket: no pendulum. I then looked in the car, and it took me half an hour to locate it in the footwell of the driver's seat. I brought the pendulum inside, cleansed it, and took it to my treatment room. The next day when I came to treat my client with it, I looked on the shelf where I'd placed it and it had vanished! I eventually found it underneath my therapy couch. However, when I dowsed over my client, it did not move; it failed to give me an indication of movement on every level and it felt heavy, lifeless, and dull as I held it in my fingers.

This taught me a valuable lesson. The lesson being to always try to connect with a crystal *before* you buy it and *never* to think that a crystal will automatically resonate with your being just because you would like it to!

I now ensure that when I do purchase a new pendulum, I attune my energy with it whilst in the shop, thus helping me make the right choice.

13

Feathered Friends

Randy the Rooster

"You *must* help," came the plea down the telephone line. As Madeline progressed with the full story that led to her cry for help, I felt that if I went ahead and agreed to an appointment, my own personal safety might be jeopardized! Madeline explained that she had hatched a Sussex cockerel, Randy, from show stock parents of excellent temperament. However, the bird in question had begun biting her and her husband, Alf, at just eleven weeks old. Madeline said that she had read about some bonding techniques for domestic birds, and had even made a sling in which to carry the cockerel around. He had mellowed slightly with this, but he was still testing boundaries.

In my years as an animal healer I had only given healing to two other cockerels, and that healing wasn't for problems associated with aggression. I just adore chickens, as I have my own Welsummer hens, so I went along to the small farm on the outskirts of Swaffham two weeks later and spied a very handsome chap pecking at the ground beside a small pond. That must be him, I thought as I sat in my car for a moment and watched him; he didn't look too scary! I was wrong. It soon became apparent that this wasn't Randy, for just as I was about to get out of my car, I heard a noise which made me jump. Madeline came running out of the farmhouse waving her arms and shouting. Apparently Randy had leapt out from under a bush to take a run at my car, only to land on the roof. After a five minute commotion, Randy flew down from the roof of my car, made a loud squawking noise, and shook himself. Just as I thought it was safe to set foot in the yard, a very arrogant Randy flew aggressively towards me. Thankfully I had my wellingtons on, so he only managed an angry peck on the rubber below my knee.

Safely inside the farmhouse, Alf made us all a welcoming cup of tea and I completed the consultation form. Randy was just over a year old and his aggressive outbursts had become worse in recent months; so much so that their six-year-old grandson, Reece, was unable to go out into the farmyard unsupervised. The situation came to a head when they had to remove Randy at night from "his girls" because he had even started to attack them by pecking at their feathers if he couldn't get to the highest roosting pole. Every night, Randy had to be picked up and taken to a separate coop; not a pleasurable task. One particular night, when Alf had put him on the floor of his individual coop, Randy had whirled around and taken a vicious bite of Alf's hand, causing an open wound. Even though he was chastised, at every opportunity he'd run at Alf and Madeline whenever their backs were turned. Lately, and because he needed to be deloused, whenever he was picked up he would bite severely.

I knew I had my work cut out for me! One thing a healer with common sense doesn't do is put their own health and safety at risk in any way, so I asked if Randy could be "contained" whilst I worked with him. Approaching his coop, I could see that he didn't like the fact that all his other feathered friends were free-ranging whilst he was caged. I placed a mat upon the ground and Randy started to run up and down the pen extremely fiercely. He then began to flap his feathers as if to warn me off, but I wasn't going to let Randy determine the outcome of the treatment. I inhaled slowly and became more and more relaxed as I did so. Madeline and Alf were seated on a bench behind me, quietly observing. Randy decided he would like to stand on one leg, and at this point I thought he was going to do other acrobatics to try to impress me or possibly warn me off.

I decided to use Reiki to heal Randy, as I could work from a short distance without actually putting myself in danger. Closing my eyes, I almost instantly felt an energy pulling me towards him. I held my hands out, facing towards him, and could feel him coming closer towards me. He lifted his head and crowed, and I opened my eyes to see Randy looking inquisitively at me with his head tilted on one side. He was by this point very close to me, though thankfully the wire separated us and kept me safe. I held out my hands again as I tried to link in with Randy, but all I kept seeing in my mind's eye was the color red; this was probably his root chakra, which, when out of balance, can indicate a problem with aggression. I channeled a soft, red-colored energy through the symbols I used, aiming to stabilize any excessive energy in this area. Randy then sat on the floor, his legs tucked under him, seemingly to get himself more comfortable, and he looked me in the eye. As I moved my palms slightly out towards him, Randy softened his gaze and then closed his eyes. I instinctively knew that he needed more healing, that he was misunderstood, and that all his antics were because he wasn't being listened to. Mind to mind, I told him I understood and could offer help.

At this point, speaking in a soft voice so as not to disturb the cockerel, I asked Madeline and Alf if they could hold out their hands and connect with Randy too, which they did. The three of us witnessed Randy move his head from side to side and then lower it so it was almost touching the ground. As I ended the session, I could feel that the energy through the wire had become calm and grounded. Madeline and Alf couldn't believe their ears as Randy let out a peculiar noise, almost like a squawk instead of crowing, and then rose to his feet. With a shake of his feathers, he stood again on one leg while he stretched out the other. Stretching is an initial sign post-treatment to indicate that the energy has been absorbed by the animal. He stood to look at me and I knew instinctively that he had released something. What the release was I will never know, but from that day forwards, Alf described the healing session as Randy having received a personality transplant!

To all our amazement, Randy never needed another healing session. Whatever it was that was troubling him seemed to have disappeared in that initial hour of healing. Three weeks later, I received a photograph of Randy and Alf mowing the lawn; Randy was perched on the seat of the mower at the side of Alf whilst he cut the grass! They became the best of friends, for reasons unknown to any of us!

Gert and Daisy-Mae

I love chickens, the larger breed varieties especially, and I vowed I would keep some hens of my own when we moved to Norfolk. I researched the breed that would be the right ones for us: docile, easy to handle, non-flighty, non-aggressive, and friendly with other animals. We chose Welsummers, and we haven't regretted it for one moment. Gert and Daisy-Mae have brought so much joy to our lives, and much life to our garden. They are certainly not placid, liking to chase pheasants, wild birds, and even our neighbors' two cats, but their antics have provided us with much mirth, especially last summer when Daisy managed to locate a dried-up frog under the gas tank. Gert snatched the dried-up old amphibian and ran around the garden as fast as she could, with wings flapping and the frog hanging from her beak, Daisy in hot pursuit!

Hens seem the ideal pet to me: friendly and full of fun, and of course they provide tasty eggs with the brightest yellow yolks for breakfast. Nothing quite beats the thrill of collecting freshly laid eggs, and seven years on I still love doing this. I don't think the novelty will ever wear off, and I can certainly see why once you keep hens, you will always keep hens.

Yet it hasn't all been plain sailing. After just six weeks of being a hen keeper, I had to give healing to Gertie. As she moved around the garden I noticed that she had a lump in her chest. After reading my hen-keeping books, I deduced this was a protruding crop (top of the esophagus) due to food impaction. I picked her up and massaged the area, which certainly seemed to help somewhat; it reduced in size after a few hours. However, after about three days I noticed that Gertie was lifting her head, opening her beak wide, and wasn't enjoying her food. The lumpy crop mass had also rotated towards the side of her chest. A vet trip was needed.

The vet confirmed that Gertie had an impacted crop and said she could operate. Gertie's crop was slit, the food removed, the residual food flushed out, and the crop sown back up again. When I brought Gertie home, I placed her on my lap and gave her hands-on healing, as well as put a quartz crystal on a shelf within the hen run. She recovered incredibly quickly. I had taken this hen's life into my care, and it's a jolly good job I did, because seven years on she's still laying beautiful, large, rich brown eggs and is a happy and healthy girl!

When I am healing one chicken that is part of a large flock, it is amazing to see all the other fowl race over towards me, often enthralled at the energy adjustments that are taking place. They are incredibly intelligent creatures and they can often solve complex problems, understand cause and effect, and also anticipate and plan for the future. Young chicks even display an understanding of object permanence. This is when an object is taken away and hidden from their view. Young chicks still know that the object exists. In humans, object permanence doesn't start to develop until a baby is about six months of age, but chicks show this incredible ability as early as two days old.

14

Animal Auras

The Tale of the Red Lady

I was about eight years old and in the city center with my grandma. We were in the queue at a market stall, about to purchase some of my granddad's favorite rum and butter toffees. As I gripped Gran's hand, I saw a red swirl of mist pass over the counter. It interwove through the sweets on top of the stall and then trailed around my grandma. I jumped as I saw it descend beneath our feet, and Gran asked me if I was okay and squeezed my hand. I said I was, and carried on watching this red mist move and swirl around the queue of customers. All of a sudden I heard a piercing cry from a young woman in the queue in front of us who, to me, looked very rotund. The red mist stopped above the woman's head, and then, almost like a shower, it surrounded the whole of her body from her head to her feet before dissipating into the floor below. It turned out that this young woman was going into labor five weeks early, and her baby was well and truly on the way. A crowd gathered around her and an ambulance quickly arrived; Gran and I made our purchases and were soon on our way home, struggling to get through the crowds of onlookers.

The Spiral Arc

I do not know whether what I saw that day at the market was the pregnant woman's aura, given how it behaved, but that experience of seeing color was one I didn't forget. Still, I didn't think much about it until my early twenties, when I became aware of the power of color after attending a mind, body, and spirit event at a local school with a couple of friends. At the fair was a Kirlian photographer, also known as an aura photographer. Kirlian photography was developed by Semyon Kirlian, who believed that through special photographic techniques he could capture the essence, or electro-magnetic field, around plants, humans, and other living matter. This radiance or energy field, which manifests in different colors, is called the aura.

I asked the photographer for a little more information about what Kirlian photography actually involves, and once I felt comfortable with the process I sat down and awaited my photograph. After it was taken, and to the astonishment of my friends and I, the photographer said that rarely had he seen such definite colors within a photograph; furthermore, he had never seen one with golden sparks almost flying from each of the shoulders. As we stared at my photograph, we were drawn in by colors of the deepest green, a majestic-looking rich purple color surrounding my head, and a white spiral arc of light sitting at the top of it.

I brought my photograph home and decided I needed to look into the auric colors more deeply. Armed with books from our village library, I found the whole subject fascinating, and was surprised to read that the auric field of a human being expands to twenty-one feet. This explained how when I stood beside certain people I got the heebie-jeebies! The whole subject of auras expanded my knowledge of healing, as I discovered how often auras are in need of healing due to all they are subjected to on a daily basis. Of course, it also triggered the memory of my experience of the red mist swirl at the market stall twenty years earlier.

As I reflected on what I had actually seen as a child, it all started to make sense. Red is associated with energy and is a base for turning plans into action; there was certainly action on that particular day at the market stall. Red is associated with the genital area, so understandably this color played its part in triggering the labor.

What Is an Aura?

Have you ever looked at a candle flame and seen not only the orange flame, but also the glow which extended outwards, way past the physical candle? This is an aura. It is a form of energy beyond the physical realm and it is said that all living things and all living objects manifest such an aura. This explains why animals, trees, rivers, and crystals all possess an energy that we resonate with.

The Energy of Auras

To see an auric field, first we need to understand the energy that creates it. We live in a vibratory universe, and although it may seem and feel solid and grounded, it is actually made up of countless minuscule atoms and molecules that are constantly in motion. It teaches us that we don't end with our skin and that there is energy to every level of our being. Even our emotions have an aura; good, bad, or indifferent.

The energy within your home has its own aura too, and you will be able to feel how energy differs in various places. For instance, your kitchen may feel livelier than your lounge. Your bathroom may not even feel like it has its own energy, yet your garden may have a spiritual or peaceful energy. You can't describe how each room feels, yet you know that each one feels different. It's the same when you walk into a room and you instinctively know when there's been an argument; you feel you could cut the energy with a knife. Each place has its own energy, its own aura.

Animal Auras

Working with auras and understanding how they relate to our animals takes a great deal of practice, but once you have built up your knowledge and experience of auras, you can clearly interpret what's really going on in their energy field.

When the Aura Becomes Affected

Think of the animal's auric field as a two-way filter between themselves and the world around them. The aura protects animals from negative external factors, helping to filter out unwanted energies; it is essential for their survival. The size and shape of an animal's aura is dependent on the size of the animal and can change depending on their overall energy levels and health. Environmental factors also play a part in determining the size of the energy field.

Things that weaken the auric field of animals:

- Poor diet/lack of nourishment

- Lack of exercise or overexertion

- Physical abuse

- Mental abuse

- Abandonment

- Sibling dysfunction

- Giving birth

- Medication

- Restriction: crates, cages, kennels

- Family unit dysfunction: divorce, separation, etc.

- Moving house

- Kennels/catteries

- Stress and anxiety

- Grief

- Lack of stimulation

- Jealousy

- Intimidation or aggression

Each situation above can lead to the animal having an irregular-shaped auric field. Its auric energy may then turn inwards, creating physical, emotional, or behavioral problems.

Cleansing the Animal Aura

It is vital to the health of the animal that the flow of energy in the energy field is free from interference or corruption from stagnant, unhealthy, and impure energies that can block its normal flow. If you have detected auric dysfunction in your animal, it may be cleared and removed using aura cleansing.

It's important to note that if you take on a rescue animal, its external energy field will possibly have many impurities and may need cleansing as soon as it comes into your home. The animal's energy may be holding on to past experiences from its previous owners—abuse, trauma, abandonment—or even negative energy from within the rescue center.

The Animal Magic Aura Cleansing Technique

This technique is performed over the whole body of the animal, as well as over individual chakras. Aura cleansing uses the hands, especially the fingers, to remove undesirable energy attachments.

Whilst performing aura cleansing, the hands are moving in a particular way. They are "drawn out" away from the body of the animal, removing any auric energy impurities through the movement. This whole action is done in a slow, deliberate manner. One must concentrate deeply during the act of aura cleansing.

Step by Step—The Animal Magic Aura Cleansing Method

Detect any areas in need of auric cleansing with a pendulum.

Place one hand palm-down, with the fingers spread a little apart, over the first area to be cleared.

Extend the fingers straight out, slightly pulled up at the tips.

The hand, at the beginning of the drawing-out motion, is about one inch above the body surface, and at the end of the motion around ten inches above the body.

The entire motion takes approximately five seconds and you are removing the impurities in one steady sweep.

While performing this motion, visualize; sense any auric impurities being removed.

As you do this, feel the energy in your hand and fingers. Feel the energy field around your fingers expanding and growing strong; sense it attracting, pulling, and clearing away any undesirable energy, drawing your hand upwards as you move onwards to the rear of the animal's body.

Remove the impurities from the patient's auric field. You may see, with physical eyes, your hand and fingers expanding and catching the undesirable energies. I can actually see this energy sticking to my fingers.

Once it's removed from the animal's body, shake your hands to discharge the impurities from yourself and wash your hands under running water.

Do the exercise above for each impurity you notice.

Note: Once any impurities are removed, they lose their charge and their ability to cling to the auric field of the patient. The impurities dissolve, become dead, and have no further effect on the animal client.

The Subtle Animal Bodies

Animals have five bodies within their aura; these are called "subtle bodies." Each subtle body is assigned a color, and they are:

- **Physical:** Red
- **Etheric:** Orange
- **Emotional:** Green
- **Mental:** Blue
- **Spiritual:** Magenta

The Animal Auric Colors

The various colors in the animal aura indicate the animal's state of health. Pay particular attention to the *etheric body* of your client, which is about three inches above their physical body. Any dark spots or stickiness may suggest a health problem. The translation of the aura colors can vary from healer to healer, as each one of us sees color differently.

Interpretation of Auric Colors

The interpretation of auric colors takes many years of practice and can only be developed through several years of healing. Over the last twenty years I have kept detailed journals, which have helped in my personal interpretation of the aura colors of the many hundreds of animal clients I have treated.

A Clear or White Aura

- High intelligence and is a quick learner
- Likes to prove their love at every opportunity, loving through adversity and retrusting easily after being severely mistreated
- A great candidate for the show or performance ring
- Usually a "one person" animal, and can be protective and watchful

- Tendency to be physically agile, sure-footed, strong, and very healthy

- Has the ability to "sense" when the environment around them is unbalanced and will act accordingly

- Tendency to be picky about food, personal cleanliness, and sleeping quarters

An Indigo or Violet Aura

- Great sensitivity and perception of sight, hearing, taste and smell; this animal may even experience a heightened sense of touch and enjoy body therapies

- Can sense other animals or humans in need, and want to reach out to them

- Has the ability to visualize and concentrate on multiple tasks

- Makes excellent "PAT" animal or a healer animal within in a nursing home environment

- Makes for a great surrogate pet

- May also be susceptible to many allergies: foods, mold, grass, etc.

- May suffer from itchy skin, rashes, or hot spots

- May be on a special diet or need to sleep on special bedding

- May prefer sleeping to going for hacks/walks

A Blue Aura

- May carry their emotions around their throats and necks; they may attempt to remove whatever is placed at the throat and dislike collars, harnesses, etc.

- A tendency to be overvocal

- Likely to be highly sensitive to your touch and/or voice

- May have special toys or blankets that they favor

- May repeat the same actions over and over with their favorite items, whether it is a toy, clothing item, or bedding

- May want to rest on or close to something with your scent on it

- Will be very attentive to your every mood, will try to move close to you at every opportunity to show that they are listening and waiting for your approval and love.

- Can be seen as quite needy animals when really they often just prefer being with you to doing anything else!

- Tend to be a little less active than other pets

- Great comforters and nurturers.

A Green Aura
- Tend to be very bright and alert

- Will demonstrate a lot of respect towards you

- Can show symptoms of being self-absorbed; can sit for hours preening, licking, or sniffing at their body or at a favorite chew toy or treat

- Gives you unconditional love, bordering sometimes on jealousy and possessiveness

- Will be picky about their tastes

- Can easily display jealous traits if you display affection towards another animal

A Yellow Aura

- Tend to be very assertive, have a strong will, are very determined, and could be stubborn

- Can be animated and may "mimic" sounds close to your own

- Will want to spend most of the day in play mode

- Tire easily of just one toy and want to move quickly on to play with another

- Very bright and energetic; learns tricks and commands easily, and then forgets them just as easily because their attention span is so short

- Can tire easily because they expend so much energy in every activity in which they engage; active one moment and asleep the next

- Eat and drink very quickly because they want to spend their time investigating new toys and adventures with few interruptions

- Can be hyperactive and like to chew a lot

- Like being the center of attention

An Orange Aura

- May pace or stamp or swish their tail a lot

- Will need a lot of space to move around

- Need a lot of activities to keep them stimulated and busy

- Constantly on the move

- Tend to display a highly sexual nature, so when around other animals of the opposite sex, will be overly attentive and sometimes engage in inappropriate behavior

- Do not like the feeling of being caged, in a stable, kennel, crate, or carrier

- May be seen as disobedient because they do not follow commands

- Most likely love to have their bellies rubbed

- Are grazers and will eat and drink when they feel the need, not at regular times

- Like to have a lot of light surrounding them, such as the sun and greenery

A Red Aura

- A very grounded animal

- Possess a lot of vitality, strength, and stamina and have great survival instincts; they are "fighters"

- Tend to use all of their natural senses, touch, smell, sight, sound, and taste, to connect with other animals and humans

- Love to be outside where they can be close to the elements and engage in natural behaviors; they like to roll, hunt, chase, and chew

- Tend to show both pleasure and displeasure with sounds: purrs, growls, barks, howls, whinnies, bobbing of their heads, clucking, etc.

- Work very hard to please their human

- Remain loyal to the end of their days

- Need a lot of fresh water and food around them, as fresh a food as possible

- May wake a lot throughout the night

Additional Information

Understanding the colors of the auric field of animals is vital when working with its energy to engage them with healing, but as I said earlier, it takes much practice to become proficient at aura detection.

Strengthening the Animal Aura

There are several things you can do to strengthen an animal's aura. For example:

- Place colored crystals at corresponding chakra points during healing
- Lay colored silk squares upon the body
- Add solarized water, which is pure mineral water that has been energized by the sun, to their drinking water
- Direct the appropriate aura color needed when healing
- Place appropriate-colored bedding, collars, or blankets etc.

15
Soul Speak
Communication

The Language of Energy

Humans have the ability to use words to express themselves, whilst animals have only their energy and body language. Animals may not speak in the vocabulary or vocal sense we are familiar with, but they can make their presence known and show their love and affection to us through the language of their energy. Animals have an amazing ability to use their body to communicate with their human companions, with other animals, and with their enemies! Just look into their eyes next time they snuggle up against you on the sofa; without words they say it all.

Foxed

On my way to a Midsummer Solstice celebration in Nottingham in 2002, the lines of soul speak communication were opened to me, but not by a cat, dog, or horse; I was lucky enough to share the private and innermost world of fox.

It was a summer's evening and my fiancé, Louis, and I were heading to the celebration, which was around twenty-five miles away from where we lived. Eight miles into our car journey, something extraordinary occurred. As we motored along the A57, my foot lifted from the accelerator; it was as though someone else was controlling not just my foot but the whole of my body.

Louis became concerned, looking over at me and asking if I was okay. I replied that I was, but I pulled over to a lay-by beside an area of woodland, where I felt an overwhelming desire to exit the car, and asked Louis to stay put. It was still light enough to see, as the late evening sun shimmered through the trees, and somehow I knew I would be safe to enter the woodland alone. Something was "calling" me and I just couldn't explain who, what, or why.

I crossed over a few fallen oak branches at the woodland's edge and stepped under the large canopy of trees. As I looked onwards, directly in front of me, not more than thirty feet away, was a majestic-looking hind; her piercing eyes looking straight through me. I was taken aback as I stood and watched her in awe. Her energy was speaking to me and I sensed all was not well, as I started to feel uneasy, and then an air of sadness and helplessness washed over me. As I moved, a branch snapped under my feet and the deer scurried deeper into the forest. Instead of returning to the car, I knew I needed to stay in close proximity to her, and she led me deeper into the trees, turning back twice to ensure I was still close by.

What had initially been a sense of joy and excitement at observing this wild creature so closely had now turned into a feeling of foreboding. The trees had become denser and I had to fight my way through the overhanging branches to see my way clear. I glanced over to my immediate left and caught a glimpse of ginger; it was a fox's tail. I was now in pursuit of a hind *and* a fox; how magical! Both deer and fox paused for a couple of moments, and I stopped suddenly as I didn't want to alarm them in any way.

The fox fixed my gaze before retreating into the brambly undergrowth. I took a few more steps before the vixen reappeared near a bank of fern, and I was amazed when I saw that sitting alongside her were three fox cubs. I was overjoyed to be witnessing this majestic sight, almost tearful, yet I still couldn't shake the sense of disharmony; I would soon discover why. My head became light and I experienced a buzzing sensation in my forehead; the fox was opening up a communication channel with me. She told me how one of her cubs had become trapped by "the people of the night" and she cried, as she was desperate not to lose another one. My sense of foreboding began to make sense. I felt blessed to receive such direct communication from this wild animal and I was honored that she trusted me enough to think that I could help her and her young.

The vixen and cubs moved away, and I could still see the hind in the distance. She looked down at the ground and then up at me. I could hear the cubs rustling in the nearby brambles as I moved towards the deer. About eight feet away from her, I witnessed such a shocking sight: two gin traps had been set on the woodland floor, both of which were wide open awaiting their next victim. How could anyone want to harm an animal in such a barbaric way, an animal in its native environment who called the woodland its home, causing harm to no one. I bent down and picked up two pieces of fallen pine, placing each one on the trap plates, snapping them shut.

I turned around as I heard Louis calling me, and as he emerged from the trees, I turned back to look at the vixen, her cubs, and the deer, but they were all nowhere to be seen. "Who was the woman you were speaking with?" asked Louis. I was puzzled, as I hadn't spoken with any woman, yet Louis insisted he heard a female voice while he was walking towards me through the trees.

As we walked back to the car together I tried to make sense of the whole event and I couldn't. The wonder of wild nature never ceases to amaze me and I am grateful for all my encounters with wild animal-kind, especially this one on the special eve of midsummer.

Saskia

The way in which animals communicate with their own kind always takes me by surprise. I am in awe of their ability to convey their emotions and all manner of things without using a single spoken word. Another such instance was when we arrived home with our puppy, Saskia, who's now eleven years old. I knew we needed to integrate a boisterous puppy carefully into the domain of our two aging house cats, Tess and Jemima, so I had decided to take two weeks off work to help things progress as smoothly as possible. The moment I stepped through the door with Saskia in one of the cat carriers, Tess and Jemima caught sight of her, and, with noses in the air and their tails down, they made a hasty retreat up the stairs.

The following day, Saskia was allowed to explore the downstairs of the house. We were having a play session on the rug in front of the fire when I heard the padding of cat footsteps coming down the stairs, and then the ginger face of Tess came peeking around the doorway. Saskia, being an inquiring puppy, ran towards Tess, who hastily retreated back up the stairs; only having little legs, Saskia could not even make the first tread to follow.

On the third day, I was in the kitchen washing the dishes and I looked into the living room. I couldn't believe my eyes; Saskia was cleaning Tess's ears! Tess absolutely adored her ears being rubbed, stroked, and cleaned. Instinctively, even as an eight-week-old puppy, Saskia knew this too, so from day three a grand bond was formed between the two of them. We called Tess and Saskia "partners in crime," as they were always hatching some sort of devilish plan together!

Initially I was quite nervous about integrating Saskia with Tess. The reason behind this was that when we adopted Tess from the Cats Protection League, she had previously lived with a family, but due to her fear of their dog she had lived in a spare bedroom for four years, never venturing out for fear of being attacked by their resident terrier. This led Tess to develop three serious health issues. She was morbidly obese; and when we adopted her she weighed twenty-three pounds, even having already shed some of the weight she arrived at the shelter with. Tess needed a special home that would endeavor to maintain her weight-loss program. Furthermore, because of the weight and lack of exercise from living in a confined space, she had developed hip dysplasia and looked rather knock-kneed! This situation had affected her on a psychological level too. She had become agoraphobic, as a few years earlier, when she had decided to venture out into her previous owners' garden, she had been attacked on her own doorstep by a neighborhood cat. Subsequently, an abscess formed that had to be surgically removed. With all of this in mind, you can see our concerns over the Saskia-Tess introduction.

Speaking of Tess: Tess never quite grasped the concept of hands-on healing. She would move as soon as I rested my hands upon her and would often look at me rather suspiciously. However, she did adore my large collection of crystals. As soon as I took the crystals from shelves to cleanse them, or dowse over the ones I should use, Tess lay straight in the middle of them, rolling over and absorbing their energy. Tess was quite a special crystal-cat, for whenever I bought new crystals to add to my kit, I'd place them on the floor and Tess would tell me whether or not they were "sleepers." Sleepers are crystals that require their healing potential to become awakened through attunement, and it takes a very spiritually aware cat to be able to detect this. Tess was really quite special.

Communication through Movement

Canines who become support dogs, such as guide dogs for the blind, communicate brilliantly in a style that not only saves lives but is unbelievably safe, reliable, and trustworthy.

Have you ever seen a sad dog in a rescue center? How do you know they're sad? Is it because their ears are flattened down, their tail is between their legs, their back is arched, or their head is hanging low? It's most likely one or all of the above. On the other hand, a tilt of the head of a happy dog wanting you to join in their fun and games, or the lifting of a paw for attention, says it all.

From their expressions to our words, it is all communication. Combined, it gives us an opportunity to understand, to reflect on, and to reward. One pat or stroke goes a long way in an animal's world. They probably understand the way we use tone of voice and spoken language to call their name better than we understand their various styles of communication.

Perceiving

To see what animals see, get down to their level nearer the ground and you become much more aware of why they see and react to things the way they do. There are flailing feet all around them, cars rushing by, bicycles ridden by loud children, and unidentifiable objects being hurled into their domain via the letter box every morning. I personally like to lie down on the floor every now and then to get a feel and sense of what my own animals are seeing. I try to imagine if I move a piece of furniture around, for instance, how this may impact behavioral changes. It's more than a simple chair being moved; it's a part of their world that has changed!

Listening to Animals

Animals communicate with us all the time, whether we are aware of it or not. It is estimated that the average human thinks around 40,000 thoughts every day, so it is little wonder that animals often receive a busy signal when they try to tune in with us.

Have you ever wondered what your animal could be thinking? Do animals feel and experience life the same way we do? As an animal communicator I have been instrumental in finding lost animals, including my own barn cat who had gone missing for five days. On the fifth day I opened up a communication trail, followed the information Muddle conveyed to me, and found him a little over a quarter of a mile away, unhurt but hiding in thick brambly undergrowth. I have also communicated with deceased pets, helped owners to understand their animals' behavioral issues, and simply facilitated more understanding, deepened love, and opened more free-flowing communication between them and their treasured companions.

Communicating with animals is an ability we are all born with. As we grow, our sense of speech takes over and we forget how to truly "listen" to others, human or animal. Our innate telepathic sense allows us to communicate our thoughts, feelings, and emotions over distance.

Tapping into the Subconscious

Soul speak communication involves tapping into a level of consciousness that allows a type of communication to occur that does not involve speech and is not conveyed through gestures or body language. Because animals do not verbalize, they communicate this way all the time with humans.

Animal-to-animal language includes:

- **Body language:** Posture, Tail, Ears, Mouth, Eyes, Feet, Head
- **Vocalization:** Barks, Howls, Whines, Whimpers
- **Scent:** Pheromones left through urination

When humans and animals have experiences, it stimulates electrical activity in the brain. This activity is measured in Hertz, or cycles per second. Meditation—quietening the mind and being present in each moment—will help you harness your ability to communicate. When we are able to master this skill, a wide variety of information becomes available.

Animals have much to communicate. Each animal is individual, with their own personality, life purpose, and soul. They have many messages for us, about their health, their past, their welfare, etc. Most animals are also blessed with intuitive powers and it's not uncommon for animals to be gifted with prophecy, as I discovered with my own cat Tansie. Soul speak communication can be a very enlightening experience, and you may well see your pet in a new light.

Tinker Top

Since those very early days of communicating with the animals who followed me to nursery school, and with Timmy my rescue cat, I have communicated with hundreds of animal clients. One memorable and moving communication session was with a client called Tinker Top.

The lilac was in full bloom as I walked through its heady scent looking for Helena's house. I'd left my car at the top of a steep, winding driveway, unsure if I'd arrived at the right property. Tinker Top was a Jack Russell Terrier, a much-loved recent addition to the family. Two days prior to my visit I'd received a very worrying voicemail message from Helena, and even though this client was out of my catchment area, being near the North Norfolk coast, I knew that I still had to try to communicate with Tinker Top.

A flustered gent, aged about sixty-five with a beetroot-red face and wild hair that protruded from either side of his hat, came running up the driveway to greet me. He introduced himself as Edward, and he was puffing on what looked like the largest pipe in the world. Edward was wearing a pair of beige checked-patterned plus fours, a collarless striped shirt with the sleeves rolled up to his elbows, and a claret paisley cravat that was neatly tucked into his shirt. He was also sporting a floppy hat with flaps on either side that hung low over his ears. This gent looked like he had stepped out from a vintage film set. At this very unfamiliar sight, others might have fled back up the driveway vowing never to return, but as he spoke he offered me a warm welcome and I immediately felt comfortable in his presence.

"Hello, hello, hello," said Edward, and as we walked down the sweeping driveway to the front door he said, "Please go through to the drawing room and I shall inform Helena of your arrival." It was all very formal, and as the house was a huge Georgian affair with tall windows, it was all in perfect symmetry.

Helena came into the room; we shared greetings and went through the consultation in relation to Tinker Top. I made written notes as I was told the moving story about how Tinker Top had taken residency within the household.

Five weeks previously, Edward had let out the other dogs for their morning run around the grounds: Thor the Great Dane and Zak, a black Labrador. Normally they would both return for their breakfast, but on this particular day Zak hadn't come back. Edward went searching for him, along with their groundsman. They searched and called out for Zak and as they moved closer to a small copse, they could hear a faint barking noise coming from the undergrowth.

As the two men cleared their way through, Zak came running out, barking frantically; they knew something was wrong. Zak led the men deeper through the trees and stood and barked beside a disturbed piece of ground. They discovered a shocking sight; a small terrier dog covered from head to tail in mud, along with a face full of cuts and scratches. As the two men took a closer look they saw the dog's right hind leg was slightly below the earth. The terrier was obviously in shock and very frightened and distressed; he tried to bark but was too hoarse and dry. The dog squealed in agony as he squirmed along the ground trying to get to his feet, but all he could do was lie there on the wet soil.

Horrifyingly, Edward noticed the ground surrounding Tinker Top was covered in blood.

Edward managed to pick up the terrified dog and wrap him in a coat. While they were carrying him back to the house, the terrier hardly had any energy left to protest; it was clear the dog was suffering and in a great deal of pain.

The vet came out the following day and said it was more than likely, judging by the cuts, marks, and old scars on Tinker Top's body, that he had been used for the barbaric act of badger baiting. The vet advised that this dog was lucky to be alive and prescribed some very strong painkillers and a course of antibiotics. He also warned Edward and Helena that it was possible that the dog might well need a leg amputation if it became infected.

With much love and care, the terrier, who Helena named Tinker Top, made great physical progress, but mentally and emotionally, Tinker Top was scarred.

In the weeks since the rescue, the dog hadn't slept through a full night. Helena explained how Tinker Top would yap and howl intermittently throughout the night, waking the other animal residents. I explained that this noise was probably Tinker Top expressing he was lonely and wanting comfort and support after his ordeal. Edward went on to tell me that Tinker Top would constantly roll over on his back whenever he saw him, despite the pain he must have been feeling in his hind leg. This, I told the couple, was a sign of submissive behavior.

I sat on the floor and edged my way across towards Tinker Top, who was looking very forlorn lying quietly in his wicker basket with his chin resting on the edge. He was predominantly white with light tan markings, and he had a lovely smudge of a deeper brown color across his nose. His ears were pulled as far back as they could get, and he sank further into his basket upon my approach. I could tell by his body language that this dog was extremely nervous and had suffered greatly.

Placing my hands on the edge of his basket, speaking softly in a comforting voice, I avoided direct eye contact. Although I meant no harm, I was aware that Tinker Top could see me as a threat and may advance to bite me. With this in mind, I did not to touch him, and I kept my gaze soft. I looked towards his chest and saw he had multiple scars across his torso and face, and a very old, deep wound on his nose. I asked Tinker Top if he would allow me to lightly touch him on his chin. Tinker Top moved his head as if to nod at me. I knew that was his way of saying that it was okay for me to touch him there.

Tinker Top was becoming calmer, and Helena left the room as she had become very emotional. My hand made contact with the front of his body, touching his scars lightly and allowing a little healing energy to be channeled.

"Can I speak to you?" came a little voice out of nowhere. "I would like to tell you what happened to me." The little voice was Tinker Top's, and I began to connect deeper with him, slowly and in his own way, allowing him to dictate the pace of the communication session. I felt the energy heighten and it was then that I realized what Tinker Top was telling me was akin to me turning the pages of a book; it was Tinker Top's own harrowing story. I moved my hands towards his heart center to open up the communication channel and my hand immediately flew back towards me. This indicated that Tinker Top had been through a very disturbing ordeal and I too became very emotional; I could feel his pain.

My hand moved over to his butterfly chakra, and it was then that his story began to unravel. I saw pictures: a time when Tinker Top had been a happy dog. He told me that he had been bought as a puppy and shared his early life with two adults and two children. When the family relationship broke down, Tinker Top, then aged about three, was taken to a rescue center. I could feel his unhappiness and the emotional pain at having the ordeal of finding a new home thrust upon him.

Tinker Top wasn't in the sanctuary for very long, as he was adopted by another young couple. However, when their first child came along, Tinker Top found himself abandoned at the side of the road, near to a lay-by. This couple obviously didn't want the commitment of a small dog and a new child, so they had dumped him. He was found roaming the roadside by two men who were exercising their terrier dogs, and they took Tinker Top home.

Tinker Top didn't settle with them, as he told me that he was kept in an outside storage area. As Tinker Top explained his surroundings, I saw in my mind's eye a corrugated hut-type building with old rusty doors and a dirty, oil-soaked floor. The feeling in my heart was very grim indeed. I saw Tinker Top catching rodents in the hut, as he was fed very little and only given food when he had "worked for it." The men taught him to dig out holes in search of badgers in woodland across the Norfolk countryside. Tinker Top told me what he had to do for these men, and at this point I had to disconnect from his energy for fear of becoming too emotional to carry on with the communication. I saw some very disturbing images of badgers suffering and being tortured in the most horrendous ways.

When I reconnected, I moved my right hand towards his butterfly chakra and the name "Sid" popped into my mind. I didn't know what this name meant, but I knew Tinker Top was so happy to be releasing some of his gruesome past.

I positioned my hands over his mid-spinal area, around his solar plexus, and I started to feel a little uneasy as anger arose within my chest. Tinker Top began to explain the events of the night he was left for dead in the copse. After Tinker Top had failed to dig out the badger from underground, the men just left him lying injured where he fell. Tinker Top had become embroiled in an attack between a badger and another dog. The men laughed at Tinker Top lying helpless as they opened a sack and placed the badger into it, and taking their other dogs, they left Tinker Top writhing in agony at the side of the badger sett.

I was so upset, as I knew that all this barbarity towards badgers involved large sums of money for betting, money gained through the sufferance of these innocent wild creatures. The badger is dug out of its sett and kept hidden to be baited later on. It is taken somewhere quiet, for example a barn, shed, or cellar, and placed into a makeshift arena, or a ring or pit from which it cannot escape. Dogs are then set upon it. Even if the badger is lucky enough to get the better of one dog, the owner may hit or otherwise injure the badger in order to "protect his pet." Ultimately, no matter how well it tries to defend itself, the badger's fate is sealed, and through injury and exhaustion, will not be able fight any longer. The baiters will then kill the badger, usually by clubbing or shooting it. Gambling is always involved, and a winning dog's value will rise, along with the price of its puppies.

I just wanted to scoop this little dog up in my arms and reassure him that everything was going to be all right, and that Helena and Edward were going to love him in the way he deserved to be loved. Given that he had suffered on both physical and emotional levels, I knew the healing of Tinker Top would not be achieved overnight.

Tinker Top let out a big sigh and a yawn, then rested his head on my hand on the rim of his basket. I knew that he'd become comfortable and content in my company.

Surrounding him in a white bubble of light, I thanked him for communicating with me. I told him that I fully understood the nature of his ordeal and assured him that the family was going to take very good care of him; that he was now safe. He raised his head and gently stretched his legs, letting out a little yelp as he was obviously still in some pain. He stood up in his basket and took a step towards me; I lowered my face and he licked my forehead. I was thrilled that we had made good progress in such a short space of time.

Tinker Top licked the air in front of my face, then retreated back into his basket, and as I ended the session I called in Helena and Edward. They both sat down around the old oak table and Tinker Top stood up and walked over to Edward. As he put down his hand, Tinker Top licked it three times and then did exactly the same with Helena. Once again Helena became very emotional, as she explained that it was the first time since his arrival that he had moved out of his basket to greet anyone entering the room. Helena asked me what I had done to Tinker Top to bring about this instant change. I said, "We've just had a chat."

I shared some of the information with this lovely couple, and it was heart-warming to watch Tinker Top lie on the top of Helena's slippers near the oven range. Even though he was just lying down he looked so much brighter, and Helena remarked how the atmosphere in the kitchen seemed clearer and lighter. Edward said that it all made so much sense as to why this little dog was taking so much time to get over his ordeal.

I mentioned the name "Sid" to Helena and she immediately burst into tears. A couple of days after finding Tinker Top, their handyman had gone into the copse to level off the disturbed ground. As he had shoveled the dirt he saw a round metal disc with the name "Sid" engraved on it; I smiled and looked towards Tinker Top.

As I rose from the table, trotting into the kitchen came Tilly, a gorgeous Persian cat, followed by three more: Purdy, Priddy, and Bliss, one by one, all in a straight line. "Do they always do everything together at once?" I asked. "They only come out of hiding when we have a *special* guest," said Edward. "I'm honored," I replied, and left them all with my love.

How to Soul Speak

Soul speak communication goes much deeper than simply understanding what an animal is thinking. It is about understanding why our animals are feeling a certain way; why, and what we can do to help them.

Mind to Mind

Throughout my work as an animal communicator, I am often asked by clients how I can read their animals' minds. I reply that I don't read minds, and this can lead to much confusion. I explain that soul speak communication is not about reading an animal's mind; it is about good listening.

Being a good listener is essential to effective communication because hearing what animals have to tell us is the first step to understanding them. We may instinctively know when Sammy wants to be let out for a run, or when Sally wants her dinner, but what about other types of communication your animal wishes to convey to you, communication that may be full of deep feeling, thoughts, past memories, experiences, and wisdom. This is the type of communication I call "soul speak." Making this sort of connection with any animal is speaking and listening, with soul.

The Bond of Communication

Anyone who shares a bond with an animal already communicates in several ways: voice, body language, and intuition. Soul speak communication is communication with an animal via a mind-to-mind process and can be likened to telepathy. Animal communicators are sometimes referred to as pet psychics or pet whisperers, yet being an animal communicator is a two-way process; there is a sender and a receiver, so in many ways we are "animal listeners."

Soul speak communication is a very natural thing to do. Some people, like me, have communicated with animals for most of their lives without even realizing it. Many children communicate with animals naturally, just as I did, until they recognize it is simply not accepted by adults. If you love an animal and feel you have a special bond, you are already tuned in but may not be processing the communication consciously or effectively.

Soul Speak = Animal Communication = Soul Listening

Reasons to soul speak:

- To strengthen the bond between you and your animal

- To help you identify which fear or negative emotion is causing your pet's illness

- To verify that any animal's fear is completely gone and the animal is safe to enter into previously fearful situations

- To help you understand reasons behind aspects of their behavior

- To help you determine and understand the life of the animal before they came to live with you

- To understand your animal's needs. This may include specific food requirements, nutrients, toys, etc., to enhance the quality of their life

- To reassure an animal who becomes anxious when they see suitcases being packed that you'll soon return hom.

- To check in with your animals while you are on holiday or a business trip, to ensure they are healthy and happy

- To let your animals know that you are on your way home from work

- To contact a lost or stolen animal and ask for descriptions of their surroundings

- To communicate with wild animals to enable an understanding of their lives

- To ask for their help in decision making and for personal guidance

Are You Communicating Already?

Take a look at the sentences below and see how many resonate with you:

- Sick, lost, or injured animals and birds seem to find their way to you.

- Your love of animals began when you were a small child and you had a range of toy or real animals that you cared for.

- When you are thinking about going out for the evening or away on holiday, your pet appears inseparable from you even before you begin preparations.

- Family members report that your pet starts waiting for you five or ten minutes before you return home.

- Other people's pets become instant friends, even if you have not met them before.

- A pet will sit close by you if you are unwell.

- Your animal growls and hisses at a stranger who subsequently proves unreliable.

- Your animal has warned you away from a potential hazard, no matter how small.

- When you speak to an animal or bird it becomes silent and still rather than becoming overexcited.

- You find you can calm animals with the power of your voice.

- You can soothe a sick or frightened animal just by stroking them.

- Wild birds come close to you when you are sitting in the garden.

- You have occasionally seen colors or flashes of light around your animal.

- You become deeply distressed by the sight of a badly treated animal.

- You donate to or support animal charities.

Communicating with Your Own Pet

There are many ways to experience soul speak communication. Among them are thoughts, emotions, images and pictures, and physical sensations. If you wish to open communication channels with your own animal, the method below will help establish your link and assist in opening the lines of communication.

You may think it is best to have your animal lying on your lap for the following communication session, but in fact it is better if you are in a different room than your animal. This is because if you are connecting with them physically, their movement can distract your concentration, and for this connection journey, you need a great deal of concentration.

Step by Step—Establishing Soul Speak

Find a room where you will not be disturbed.

Allow your mind and body to relax and breathe into every stiff place in your body, breathing out any tension.

Close your eyes and allow your energy to settle in your head.

What can you hear?

What can you smell?

What can you sense?

Become aware of all you are experiencing. These are your senses awakening.

Now move your attention to the center of your chest, to your heart chakra.

Allow yourself to focus on this area and feel its energy: how does it feel? Allow yourself to experience your heart energy. This is the energy your animal senses all the time.

When you feel the connection to your heart energy, create a green bridge of light between yourself and your animal. Send love from your heart chakra to theirs and allow their love to enter yours. Can you feel their energy connecting with yours?

When you are ready, send the following thought link to them: "Thank you for sharing your life with me," or "Thank you for coming into my life."

Allow the energy from your heart chakra to rise up to your throat chakra. The throat chakra is key to all soul speak communication.

Allow yourself to feel a bright blue light pulsating and swirling in your throat chakra.

Allow this blue light to create a bridge to your animal's throat chakra, then back to yours; feel this circuit of blue energy.

Now allow the blue light to rise up to the center of your forehead, your third eye chakra, and merge the blue light with a purple light. Your third eye chakra enhances all intuitive communication.

Allow this purple light to flow towards your animal's third eye chakra and back to yours; feel this bridge of purple energy.

What can you feel? Allow yourself to *experience*.

Are you receiving a message from the energy of your animal? Allow yourself to receive.

Now feel the whole energy expanding into your ears and listen. Can you hear any message from your animal? Allow yourself to receive.

As you explore the message, the energy, and the sensations, allow your animal's energy to return back home, to their heart center.

Sense and feel how magnificent and beautiful you are. This is the part of yourself that animals see and feel all the time. Allow yourself to feel the love for you that your animal feels.

Now take three deep breaths and gently bring your awareness back to your physical body and, when you are ready, slowly open your eyes.

How Dogs Learn from Body Language

Your dog's basic body language and communication skills are instinctual, and are honed through interaction with the mother, littermates, and the humans in his early environment. A dog who is lacking in these essential skills is likely to be either shunned or attacked by other dogs. As dogs are social creatures, they quickly figure out which behaviors and signals are most rewarding, and then repeat these. They learn through observation and the direct experience of trial and error.

A dog who has been removed too early from the litter doesn't have the opportunity to develop social skills and an in-depth understanding of canine body language. This can ultimately be dangerous for him, as he may be unable to interpret the intentions of other dogs, or may use inappropriate body language that sparks hostility in them.

In their relationships with us, we have a profound effect on their nonverbal displays. Rewards for using particular signals are likely to reinforce those signals, and punishment can cause them to be suppressed. We can use this to our advantage by responding positively to calm body language. Our approval means a great deal to our dogs, so they will continue to use signals which have brought rewards in the form of affection, a game, or food treats. However, dogs who have been punished for showing signs of irritation, discomfort, or anger through growling soon learn that giving a growl leads to pain. In order to avoid this, they may suppress the warning growl and move straight into the bite instead.

Because of the long association between humans and dogs, your dog's brain is hardwired with the ability to observe and act on your body language. They may not understand the reasons for your feelings, but they can pick up the signals that reveal whether you are happy, sad, frightened, angry, or playful. If two people are arguing, the dog in the room will take one of three options to deal with the situation. The dog may remove himself as far away as possible to escape the conflict, or may try to move in between you in order to separate you ("splitting up"), or may growl at or challenge the person they view as attacking the human they are most strongly bonded to. When you are relaxed, your dog is more likely to relax.

16
Bach Remedies

O n the 24th of September in 1886, in a village called Moseley near
Birmingham, England, a holistic health pioneer was born. His
name was Edward Bach and he would later become a doctor, special-
izing in the healing power of plant medicine.

Bach was a medical student at the University College Hospital in
London and later practiced for twenty-plus years as a Harley Street
bacteriologist and pathologist. His immunology research evolved
into homeopathic research, leading to the development of seven bacterial nosodes (a nosode is best described as "a preparation of substances secreted in the course of a disease, used in the treatment of
that disease."[14]) Dr. Bach later replaced his seven nosodes with natural
herbs; this led him to discover the first of the Bach flower remedies that
we know today: Clematis, Impatiens, and Mimulus.

Bach was positive that a new system of medicine could be developed from the realm of nature, and so he took up residency in Wales. In
spring and summer he pursued new herbal remedies, treating patients

---

14   https://en.oxforddictionaries.com/definition/nosode

in the wintertime. He discovered his first twelve remedies by 1932, and a year later began making a second group of remedies: the seven helpers. In 1934, he moved to Oxfordshire; he found nineteen more remedies, which completed the Bach flower series.

Evidence suggests that humans have relied on medicinal plants since the beginning; archaeological excavations from sixty thousand years ago have uncovered the remnants of cannabis, opium poppies, and ephedra.[15] Plants and herbs have been used the world over in the effort to prevent or treat disease, and this form of medicine has been given various names—among them aromatherapy, homeopathy, floratherapy, alternative medicine, and herbal therapy.[16] Bach flower remedies fall within all of the above.

Using Bach Remedies with Animals

I am a strong believer in Bach's theory that illness is the effect of disharmony between body and mind, and that symptoms of illness can be the external expression of negative emotional states. But just as the human psyche has different states of negative being, or negative attitudes, animals also experience these states. If you look closely, you may learn how you or your animal may have experienced one or more of Bach's seven negative states of being: fear, uncertainty, insufficient interest in present moment, loneliness, oversensitivity, despondency and despair, and overcare of others.

It is important to note that Bach flower remedies work on emotional and mental levels and do not seek to cure any physical ailments. They are categorized as "vibrational" complementary medicine. They

---

15   Dennis McKenna, "How Long Have Humans Used Botanicals," Center for Spirituality and Healing's Taking Charge of Your Health & Wellbeing website, University of Minnesota, https://www.takingcharge.csh.umn.edu/how-long-have-humans-used-botanicals.

16   "Plants that Heal," Sandbox Networks, Inc., publishing as Infoplease, https://www.infoplease.com/science-health/life-science/plants-heal.

are powerful yet gentle healing tools that can catalyze the resolution of deep emotional imbalances but do not appear to have direct effects on the physical body or physical symptoms.

Bach flower remedies can be used by anyone, as they are readily available at health food stores. To use them with animals does take a great deal of research because, as discussed just above, they are used to address emotional issues rather than to directly treat physical illness. If you are interesting in formulating and creating your own flower remedies rather than purchasing them, you must undertake a recognized and professional training course in the subject, because creating these essences is not as simple as it may appear, and if they are not produced correctly, the essences can become spoiled by bacterial and mold growth, which in turn can cause further illness.

Animal Self-Medicating

Many years ago, I read a book titled *Wild Health* by Cindy Engel. Engel described parallels between animals and humans in relation to medication, and through research observed how animals knew when a certain plant material was good for them or would bring healing benefits. In fact, early humans' ideas about the healing powers of plants could have come from watching animals use them.[17]

The desire to self-medicate has been identified in animals ranging from elephants in Kenya to macaws in Brazil to domestic dogs and cats. For example, although eating grass will make them sick, dogs and cats are known to search it out; they aren't able to digest grass, lacking the enzymes, and they've learned that getting sick will relieve them of stomach aches and discomfort. Red and green macaws treat digestion issues by eating kaolin to "detoxify." Chimpanzees have been known to induce vomiting by eating particular bushes, and also have been observed eating very large quantities of Aspilia plant leaves—the leaves contain

---

17   McKenna, "How Long Have Humans Used Botanicals."

thiarubrine-A, which kills certain intestinal parasites, and the rough-
ness can act like "sandpaper" to physically remove the parasites.[18]

Humans have been involved for thousands of years with medicinal plants because we have self-medicated for centuries. Our ancestors didn't rely on a prescription from their GP in order to get well,
because there weren't doctors as we know of today. The inner wisdom
that resulted from this global experimentation is a large part of our history of healing and modern healthcare. Many modern medicines are
derived from plant bases—for example, aspirin and the willow tree's
salicylic acid.

Plant Spirit Essence

As ethnobotanist Dennis McKenna has observed, our awareness of a
plant's healing potential is related to the practice of shamanism, a religion still practiced in many parts of the world that involves a sort of
spirit medicine. Intuitive healers are able to connect, in special conditions, with the spirit of the plant; there are some plants regarded as
"plant teachers," from whom the shaman can glean information about
other plants and their healing properties.

There was traditionally a belief that the "vital spirit" of the plant was
essential to its medicinal nature, but when scientists isolated morphine
from opium in the early nineteenth century, researchers (especially in
the West) came to believe that a single and nonliving compound was
the source of a plant's curative effect, removing the thought that the
whole essence/spirit of the plant itself was responsible.[19]

---

18   "How Animals Self Medicate," DailyMail.com, https://www.dailymail.
co.uk/sciencetech/article-2868348/Do-animals-SELF-MEDICATE-Dogs-
elephants-chimps-parrots-use-natural-remedies-treat-digestive-problems-
induce-birth.html.

19   McKenna, "How Long Have Humans Used Botanicals."

The Difference between Herbalism and Flower Essences

There is no competition between herbalism and flower essences. This is because they are different modalities and work to heal in very different ways. Both herbs and essences, if made as a tincture, usually come in glass bottles with an attached dropper or pipette; however, they are very different in the way they work. In herbal tinctures, part of the plant is contained within the fluid in the bottle, because herbal tinctures are made using fresh or dried plant materials; they can also be labeled as "herbal extracts." Liquid herbal tinctures are concentrated forms of medicinal herbs that contain the beneficial properties of the herb extracted into a liquid. Tinctures are typically made by placing the relevant herb or herbs in a natural solvent, such as alcohol, glycerine, or vinegar, and allowing the mixture to infuse for three weeks or longer. The amounts of herb, solvent, and water used are very specific and dependent upon the type of herb being used. In short, tinctures contain the actual herb which could, in certain circumstances, react with any prescription medication.

The active ingredient in a flower remedy, on the other hand, is the "energy signature" from the plant, not the actual plant's physical substance like with herbal tinctures mentioned above. Subsequently, flower essences will not usually interfere with the physical action of other medicine. Nor will prescription medicine prohibit the Bach remedy from working.

The only point of caution concerns the alcohol used to bottle and preserve flower essence remedies. This can usually be ignored, as the amount of alcohol in a single dose is minute, but it's always advisable to speak with the vet if you are concerned. However, flower essences do not need to be administered orally and can work equally as well in the energy field of the animal, or by applying it to the animal's ears or paws. This is often useful when an animal is recovering from surgery, or aggressive. Mixing a little of the essence with water, placing it in a spritzing bottle, and spraying it in the environment is a great option in these circumstances.

The Fighting Felines

I had been booked to treat two cats: Dylan and Daisy. Both were rescue cats, each from traumatic circumstances. Dylan had been taken to the vet to be put to sleep after the breakdown of a marriage; he was just three years old, and as the owner no longer wanted him, he was fed irregular meals and became emaciated. Daisy had been found as a stray, scrounging for food on the local refuse site.

Hazel had taken the two cats into her home within three days of each other, but their settling-in time had not been harmonious. Both cats were soiling all around the house, but more so Dylan. Dylan was also attacking Daisy every time she entered the kitchen at meal times, and each time Hazel went to stroke her. Daisy then fled to the under-stairs cupboard and refused to come out.

Cat ownership wasn't proving to be a pleasurable experience for Hazel; when she telephoned me I could tell she was at the end of her tether. We discussed treatment options, and as Hazel had personally experienced such positive results from using the Bach Rescue Remedy to help calm her nerves for a recent driving test, she opted for using Bach flower remedies to treat both cats.

Feline Aggression

There are many reasons why cats exhibit aggression towards one another, but in this case, after completing a detailed consultation form, we had identified that in the case of Dylan and Daisy, it was territorial aggression.

Territorial aggression between cats who live with each other usually develops incrementally, but in this case, both cats had come to Hazel's house almost simultaneously, each coming from undesirable situations and neither having spent time in each other's company prior to living with Hazel.

In territorial aggression, one cat is usually the aggressor and the other the "victim." In this case, the victim was poor Daisy.

Territorial aggression incidents begin with hissing and growling and escalate to swatting, chasing, constant pursuits, and ultimately attacks and fighting; exactly what Dylan was displaying towards Daisy. Victims may become more and more intimidated by the aggressor and get defensive, hiding in nooks around the house and coming out only at times when the aggressor cat is not around. This was certainly the case with Hazel's cats, except that poor Daisy refused point blank to come out from the under-stairs cupboard at all!

With territorial aggression issues, litter tray problems can occur because the fearful cat is too afraid to move from its hiding place, hence the carpet soiling from Daisy and the territorial over-marking from Dylan.

Without any method of holistic treatment being selected and implemented, along with understanding, patience, and perseverance, territorial aggression is rarely treated successfully. Despite new behavioral procedures that are recommended and even new drug therapies that are attempted, sometimes the last solution for this problem could be to find one of the cats a new home. Hazel was willing to try her very best for each cat and, between us, we succeeded.

Keep in mind that even if a cat is aggressive with another that it lives with, this does not mean that the cat will be aggressive towards people. These felines can be lovely pets if there are no other cats present in their home. Also, restricting cats to separate areas of the household to avoid encounters can work.

Another thing to bear in mind, if you're around cats that are aggressive towards each other, is not to interfere with them, since a cat that is feeling aggressive or frightened can bite. A territorially aggressive feline might even attack an owner who has recently touched or held another cat.[20]

Finding Resolution

Hazel made it clear that she did not want either cat to be separate from the other and hoped to find a solution. We completed a detailed consultation covering how each cat had come into Hazel's care, but, as is so often the case with rescued animals, we were unable to establish much about their formative years.

We did, however, uncover specific keywords during our consultation:

- **Intolerance:** They were intolerant of each other and *possibly* their new location.

- **Fear:** Daisy was fearful of Dylan, hiding under the stairs.

- **Territorial:** Dylan was mostly soiling to mark territory, and Daisy soiling possibly out of fear.

- **Trauma:** Both cats had experienced this.

I was mindful not to overwhelm each cat, as it was their initial treatment, so I chose just four Bach remedies. Unlike other forms of healing, where trust is the main focus of the energy rather than a specific result being the focus, Bach Flower Remedy application does have its emphasis on the desired outcome. For Dylan, I used the misting application of the essences. For Daisy, I applied it to her ears.

For the initial treatment session for Dylan, I chose to utilize beech. According to Bach, beech is for those animals who need to see more beauty in all that surrounds them. Although much appears to be wrong, it can stimulate the ability to see the good growing within and without,

---

20   For a detailed discussion of territorial aggression, see Victoria L. Voith and Peter L. Borchelt, "Understanding Aggression in Household Cats," Animal Humane Society, http://www.minneapolismn.gov/www/groups/public/@ regservices/documents/webcontent/wcms1q-074018.pdf.

surrounding each situation. It helps animals to become more tolerant, lenient, and understanding. Keywords for beech include intolerance, critical tendencies, and lack of compassion. Desired outcome: tolerance.

I also chose chicory for Dylan. Chicory aids relief of possessiveness and obsessive behaviors, such as clinging, attention-seeking, and soiling for territorial marking. Chicory will help animals that won't let their owner out of sight, and constant following, or those who sulk when they can't get their own way. It is beneficial for animals who are destructive, dirty, and noisy when left alone. Chicory helps pets who are overprotective and will perform acts of nuisance such as barking, limping, biting, swatting, nipping, or vomiting whenever the owner tries to leave them. Keywords for Chicory include obsessive behavior, insecurity, and nuisance behavior. Desired outcome: accepting with confidence.

Star of Bethlehem

Star of Bethlehem, which I gave to Daisy, is suitable for those animals in great distress, or in situations which produce great unhappiness: the shock of a changing environment, the loss of their human companion, the fright following an accident, etc. Star of Bethlehem can be used for general, mental, or physical shock. This remedy is also helpful for cats that lose urine/bowel control due to emotional upset and can also be beneficial for separation anxiety. Keywords for Star of Bethlehem include distress, accident and fright, and changing situations. Desired outcome: to provide comfort and consolation.

Rescue Remedy

Bach named his emergency combination of remedies "Rescue Remedy." It combines five other remedies: Star of Bethlehem, Clematis, Impatiens, Cherry Plum, and Rock Rose. It can be used in cases of emergency or merely for everyday stress. Since Hazel's cats were experiencing the whole range, Rescue Remedy was necessary in this particular situation.

I visited Dylan and Daisy just three times over a period of five weeks, and I was astounded at their progress. They had become not just tolerant of each other but were actually able to sleep and eat in the same room, without Dylan launching into a full-blown attack on Daisy.

Hazel informed me that each cat had now taken to sleeping on one corner of the bed and each had their own separate blanket. Not once had Daisy hidden in the under-stairs cupboard and nor had Dylan lifted his paw to Daisy.

I was thoroughly pleased with the outcome and trusting the energy signatures of these simple plant essences.

17

Arbor Essentia

Arbor Essentia is a healing system I developed, based in vibrational therapy, that utilizes essences created from the arboreal world—in other words, tree essences. Each specific tree essence vibrates to a letter from the ancient Celtic Ogham alphabet. The system also incorporates specific healing tools to detect and balance a client's energy. I assess the particular essence needs of an animal client through a detailed consultation with their caretaker, then use a variety of healing tools like crystal wands, meridian balancers, dowsing implements, and tuning forks for energy detection. The Arbor Essentia method aims to provide emotional well-being, soul development, and mind-body health.

Arbor Essentia essences cannot as yet be purchased; I offer the discussion here in light of its contribution to holistic animal health care and wellness programs. Animal Essentia (Arbor Essentia as approved to be taught at the animal level) is what I call the separate animal therapy modality; practitioners can adopt it after completing my training course as part of an overall program in animal health enhancement, either in a professional practice or within a home-care setting.

Each Arbor Essentia tree essence has its own unique healing purpose. It took me more than seven years to discover each tree's unique vibration and healing ability and to develop this into my system. I spoke with every tree, I meditated with them, I reached out to them, I held my hands upon them, climbed them, pressed upon them, smelled them, sighed with them, stepped upon them, absorbed them, listened to them, and spoke with them; I actually asked questions! I listened for their answers, which took many years to find me, but I allowed my heart and soul to connect to this woodland world and I then began to understand their language.

I suppose that in a way, I connect with the tree kingdom as I do with people. I notice the profound differences between them, even ones from the same species. I notice how they move differently in the wind, and how each tree had different characteristics. Some are even scarred, just like humans and animals. I notice their twigs: some are slender, some wide, smooth, or hairy. Their branches: spotty and ridged, some of unusual color. I notice bud scars where last year's leaves have fallen. I notice face patterns unique to each species. I observe the differences in their leaves and how they sound when rustled by the breeze in autumn.

The Trees of Ogham

The Ogham, pronounced "oh-wam," was initially an ancient Celtic alphabet consisting of twenty letters, each one associated with a different tree. The word "Druid" is actually derived from the word *duir*, which has within its meaning the word "oak." It is believed that this ancient system was a Celtic tool for communication, magic, and ritual.

Unlike most other alphabets, the Ogham does not have individual characters but sets of five letters depicted by one, two, three, four, or five lines above, below, or through a base line, which is called a "druim." Every one of the Ogham letters have correspondences associated with them. With each letter, there will be typical associations: its name, symbol, tree, spiritual healing aspects, crystals, colors, affirmations, and flower essences.

Because each of the Ogham letters connects directly to a native British tree, this makes the whole system of Arbor Essentia a little more uniquely soul-connecting, I believe, than many other plant essence modalities; when I'm using a particular essence, I lay the corresponding Ogham letter, which is carved into a part of its tree (an Ogham stick), across my palm and send healing through the Ogham.

Animal Essentia

Animals, of course, have no preconceived ideas about how essences should work. They don't, for instance, think, "I have my doubts; I believe the Oak Arbor Essentia remedy would be a better option for me than Silver Birch." They merely accept the treatment without any expectations of the outcome. Animals are free from mental blocks, doubt, skepticism, placebo effects, and a myriad of mental interferences, unlike us human beings. Animals respond even more positively than humans do to Arbor Essentia, and because of the way animals accept healing, we see little miracles happen on all levels of their well-being.

Arbor Essentia and Its Vibrational Action

Arbor Essentia essences are *vibrational* in nature. They are highly diluted essences from a physical point of view, but have subtle power as potentized substances, embodying the specific energetic patterns of each tree. Similar to Bach flower remedies, their healing impact does not derive from any direct biochemical interaction within the physiology of the animal's body. Rather, these tree essences work through the various animal energy fields, and can influence an animal's mental, emotional, and physical well-being.

Arbor Essentia and Resonance

The action of Arbor Essentia can be compared to the effects that human beings experience when hearing a particularly moving piece of music, or seeing an inspirational work of art. The light or sound waves that reach our senses may evoke profound feelings deep in our soul, which indirectly affect our breathing, our pulse rate, and other physical states. These patterns do not impact us by direct physical or chemical intervention in our bodies. Rather, it is the contour and arrangement of the light or sound that awakens experience within our own soul. This is the phenomenon of resonance. In a similar way, the specific structure and shape of the life forces conveyed by each tree essence resonate with, and awaken, particular qualities within the animal's soul.

Animals are sadly all too often taken to rescue centers and euthanized for simply being misunderstood. Their owners have failed to fully understand their behavior, from the dog who barks incessantly to the cat who soils and sprays. Arbor Essentia represents a loving, healing, and beneficial animal therapy suitable for all animals. Arbor Essentia is a completely safe, nontoxic, and gentle yet powerful holistic animal therapy.

Arbor Essentia for the Healing of All Animals

My system of Arbor Essentia was designed to assist at every stage of an animal's development: birth and bonding, spaying and neutering, training, aging, and the transition from this life. It also becomes an invaluable aid during times of uncertainty, such as traveling, changing residences, adjusting to other animals coming into their lives, or indeed grieving the loss of a companion.

Animals that come from abusive or neglectful backgrounds, as many animals often do, require assistance to clear negative past patterning. With the use of the appropriate essence(s), the memory of deep despair can be relieved and the animal can move forward in life with joy and positivity.

Sensitively chosen tree essences can produce profound and lasting changes in an animal's behavior too. These changes are significant because they cannot be attributed to the placebo effect. Animals have souls, emotions, feelings, and karmic influences that affect their health and well-being, just as humans do, and these areas can be easily influenced by using Arbor Essentia.

Trixie

My first experience of utilizing my wonderful noninvasive system of Arbor Essentia healing was in 2007, with a fifteen-year-old cat named Trixie. Trixie had been rescued from a maisonette in Derbyshire when her owner, a woman of ninety-two, had passed away. Trixie found herself abandoned, alone, and desperately hungry after not being fed for days. The council had cleared out the old woman's apartment, not taking into account the lonely cat that was in the middle of it all wondering what was going on. I can't begin to imagine what thoughts were going round in Trixie's mind as she saw the skip being piled high with her owner's belongings; even Trixie's cat bed had been thrown on top. A neighbor alerted the RSPCA to Trixie's abandonment, but they were unable to help at that time, so the neighbor had no option but to take Trixie into her home on a temporary basis. A space became available at a local cat shelter, so Trixie went there until she was well enough to be rehomed. It transpired after a veterinary check-up that Trixie was FeLV positive. FeLV is a leukemia virus, so not only was Trixie going to struggle to find a forever home at the age of fifteen, she also had a virus which could potentially affect any other healthy, unvaccinated cats.

Trixie was finding it hard to cope being surrounded by all the other shelter residents, and she quickly became very withdrawn. Her health began to suffer and she gave up eating; her condition becoming so serious that she had to be fed intravenously. I was contacted and agreed to go and see Trixie at her foster home eleven miles away. What a pitiful little sight I was met with as I went through to the lounge. Trixie was lying on an old rocking chair, at her side a child's teddy bear. Judith, Trixie's caretaker, told me that she had barely moved in the nine days since her arrival. I approached the tiny cat with stealth, as I didn't want to alarm her in any way, and sat beside the chair stroking her frail body. In just seven weeks she had lost five pounds in weight; a dramatic loss for a cat already suffering from an immunodeficiency virus. I knew I needed to choose an Arbor Essentia remedy that was going to be quickly assimilated. I also decided that a combination of remedies was going to be needed, yet I didn't want to bombard Trixie with too much, too soon.

Looking into Trixie's eyes, I sensed such great loss and a total lack of interest in life. I felt sad, but I couldn't allow this to get in the way of giving healing to this listless tabby cat. I placed one drop of several Arbor Essentia essences into my palms, and it was obvious when I held them under Trixie's nose that she preferred the elm essence. Another drop of the essence on my palm, a deep grounding breath, and I placed my hands over her spine. At first I didn't physically touch Trixie, but as she started to purr, her back rose up to meet my hands. I knew then that she was asking me to make physical contact, and as I touched her frail little body, she started to make tiny head movements. Judith's face became puzzled and she quietly told me that she hadn't seen Trixie look so relaxed in the time she'd had her. I moved my hands up and down Trixie's body, moving them just a few millimeters at a time. Trixie's purr grew louder and Judith told me she had never heard her purr before now either. I placed two drops of Apple and another one of Elm onto my palms and placed my hands either side of Trixie's body, touching each side of her butterfly chakra. Trixie's purr increased in volume and so did her body! Where before she was hunched over, her neck became lengthened, her tail swished, and she did the usual cat stretch. She then meowed (something which Judith said she hadn't done since her arrival), jumped down, and walked straight up to her empty dish demanding food. The change in her with these two essences was so dramatic that I couldn't hold back my tears, nor could Judith. We hugged each other before Judith replenished Trixie's food and she proceeded to eat her meal with gusto.

Two weeks later, Judith called me to say that Trixie had now been renamed "Little Miracle" because of the dramatic improvement she had shown. Furthermore, Judith was now offering her a forever home. I am in awe of the healing power of trees.

An Unusual Case Study in Arbor Essentia

Mrs. Adams was having trouble coping with her son Ivan's iguana since he'd left for university, but she expressed skepticism about hands-on healing. I decided to implement a program of Arbor Essentia. Osiris was an antisocial four-year-old iguana who was having trouble adjusting to his new owner along with his new surroundings. Osiris was very shy and resisted handling by Mrs. Adams; he hid underneath anything he could in his vivarium to avoid her clutches. Despite his new owner being patient with him, Osiris wouldn't let her get close. He would make hissing noises and snap at her when she tried to stroke him or get close enough to offer him something to eat.

From a lengthy consultation I knew the key factors in his behavior were attributable to change, dietary habits, and his general living conditions. After pendulum dowsing to detect the main imbalance of energy, I was able to administer the Arbor Essentia essence called Ruis.

Ruis is the essence of the elder tree and promotes positive energy when there is birth or death. It was obvious that Osiris was at the end of one chapter in life and starting with a brand-new phase. In Arbor Essentia, Ruis can also be used at the beginning of any session that involves dealing with deeply embedded issues that might cause fear, or deep emotional or physical pain when treated; it will help the animal to cope with the behavioral or emotional symptoms and enable them to move forwards.

Ruis also promotes compassion and stimulates the ability to trust others, something Osiris needed to harness with Mrs. Adams. In addition, Ruis calms in situations of changeable life events and promotes unity, which both parties required in order to progress further with their relationship.

After just two Arbor Essentia treatments, Mrs. Adams saw a major transformation in Osiris's behavior. He'd started to eat regularly and even allowed her to handle him several times a day without becoming aggressive.

Ivan came home at term end, but when it came round for Ivan to return to university, Osiris wasn't fazed at all and continued to strengthen his bond with Mrs. Adams.

The Tools and Application of Arbor Essentia

In Arbor Essentia, we use a variety of tools, including the pendulum and the Ikin bobber, both of which detect energetic imbalances. These tools also help interpret the emotional state of the animal, how responsive they are to the essence, if a treatment needs to be adjusted, how successful Arbor Essentia has been post-treatment, and in what way the animal needs to be grounded after a session.

Arbor Essentia essences are quite effective when absorbed through the skin in topical applications; however, just being within the proximity of a bottle of one of the essences can have an effect. There are many creative and effective ways to use the system with animals, which include directly applying it to the skin/fur/feathers/scales; applying it as a mist and in the auric field (we do not spray any essence towards a nervous animal); on bedding, leads, collars, saddles, etc.; or applied on the animal's food.

18

Heavenly Paws

Have you ever been so connected to an animal that when it has passed over to spirit, you still feel its presence around you? This presence is an imprint of its physical being. Ties that we have with our animals cannot be cut once they depart from our lives in a physical sense. Their cord remains strong and their energy never leaves us. As such, grieving their loss can be every bit as hard, yet as necessary, as grieving the loss of a human loved one.

Life Flow

For hundreds of years, science has considered animals to be lower on the evolutionary scale. In other words, that animals have less complex brains, and are therefore incapable of the thoughts, feelings, purposes, and creativity of humankind. Research in more modern times, of course, has illustrated that animals often have complex languages of their own, great emotional potential, and thought processes similar to humans.

When people divorce themselves from a connection with nature and animals, and become separate from the spiritual essence that flows through all of life, their relationship with their fellow creatures can take on a shallow character. Without a spiritual connection to animals, even when we profess love for our "pets," we may expect the animals to supply the emotional and spiritual sustenance we are lacking within ourselves.

How different our relationships become when our domestic animal friends are viewed as equal spiritual beings, ones who are allowed to live their own lives and express their own dignity while still enjoying a mutual companionship with us and their own kind. I regard my own animals as intelligent individuals in their own right. I don't "train" them to perform tasks in order to make me feel like I've achieved something, nor do I expect anything from them. I simply respect who they are, individually and spiritually, be it cat, dog, or chicken.

Animal = Life Essence

The Latin word *anima*, which we can see within the word "animal," is variously translated as soul, spirit, breath, or life essence. Animals are whole, individual beings with their own divinity, spirituality, rights, requirements, and expressions. They feel totally connected with their human family. We listen to each other, and are both constantly changing and progressing in ways that enhance our mutual growth and understanding.

Yes, animals are different from humans. Their bodies are different, and there are vast differences in their genetic background, their functioning, and their senses; animals therefore experience the world differently than humans do. Animals as individuals combine their physical species' traits with their mental and spiritual qualities to uniquely express themselves and their purpose in this universe. While it's an advantage to study animal biology and behavior to learn about species-specific needs and patterns, this will not provide a complete understanding of animals' individual personalities, ideas, hopes, purposes, and spirituality. We can't separate the physical body from the spiritual aspect of a living being. Where there is life, there is spirit.

Spiritual connection between animals and humans involves tapping into and sharing each other's worlds or unique expressions of life. There is no need for categories and hierarchies that separate and cause condescension or alienation because we are different from each other. We merely celebrate the experience of our differences, and rejoice in the feeling of oneness in essential connection. This connection turns the key for learning from one another, sharing wisdom, and growing together in harmony.

When we slow down and tune in to our pet, we become much more aware of the nature of life around us. We observe the behavior, habits, feelings, energies, and the spirit or essence of that animal. While we each may be very different in form and function in the whole ecosystem, we all are intelligent, perceptive, uniquely vital, and part of the same spirit.

Ancient and modern tribal people recognized the need for humans to remember and focus on their deep connection to all of life and spirit, through ceremonial observance of the seasons and stages of life, and prayers and rituals for guidance and protection in their earthly ceremonies, just as I do as a Druid. The ancients regularly acknowledged that the parting in physical form does not signal the end of the spiritual aspect of life; they held passing-to-spirit ceremonies and made a big deal of death! Life goes on after death. The spiritual link cannot ever be broken, and someone who has loved an animal deeply knows this more than anyone.

Sophie

Losing Sophie, my black-and-white rescue cat, in the early 1990s was the first animal loss of my adult life. I was devastated, and I struggled to come to terms with the loss of my wonderful soul companion. I just didn't know how I was going to cope. I laid Sophie to rest under a beautiful fragile fern in the garden, beside a brick-built store where she liked to lie. The night of her passing I went to bed and wept, struggling with my loss. In the early hours of the morning, I was awoken suddenly by a thudding noise. When I turned on the bedside light, I saw a distinct imprint in the duvet. As I gathered my senses and looked closer, I saw it was cat-shaped and it was warm to the touch. It was the exact place where Sophie liked to sleep; I knew she had come to say goodbye. I slept with her photograph under my pillow, and every morning for about two weeks I woke to find Sophie's imprint beside me, until one day it wasn't there. I knew then that she had left for spirit; she had joined Timmy at Rainbow Bridge and her spirit was free.

The subject of animals in spirit surfaces time and time again with students on my training courses. They tell me how they too have shared similar spiritual experiences with their own animals. Such experiences can provide us with a great deal of comfort, knowing that our animal's energy imprint will live on forever, and will never be disconnected just because they are not physically with us.

Step by Step—Connecting with Your Animal in Spirit

During the course of my work I am often asked to communicate with animals that have passed over to Rainbow Bridge. Their owners may wish to know that they are safe, secure, or are being looked after by other animal family members that have passed before. Often, such people may ask me if their animals forgive them for being "let go" to spirit, even though we did the right thing for them by ending their suffering.

We all need to know our animals are not in any pain, are not suffering from stress, and aren't in fear. The following exercise may bring you comfort and peace of mind if you are struggling with the death of an animal.

Obtain a photograph of your animal in spirit and place it in front of you. Take three deep breaths and allow yourself to relax and your mind to let go of any unnecessary or intrusive thoughts.

Place your hands around the photograph and allow your energy to be drawn into the picture. Soften your gaze and look deeply into the photograph. Often, when you look for a while, you begin to see beyond the physical body. If you look closely enough you may see a white light, or even colors surrounding your animal. This light is their spiritual imprint, which is often left with us when they transcend the physical plane to spirit. What do you see?

Move each hand lightly across the photograph. What can you feel? Can you feel any physical sensations within your own body?

Now close your eyes. What can you see with your *inner* eyes? Does a part of the animal's body come into view? Take another deep breath and begin to listen. What can you hear?

Take another breath, and place one hand over your heart center and the other hand over the photograph. Allow yourself to feel the energy of your heart center flow into your animal. Allow yourself to feel totally connected in this moment. Share your energy, connect, feel, and send love.

Whenever you feel ready, take a deep breath, concentrate on your own heartbeat, and bring your awareness back to your physical body. Disconnect by covering the photograph with both hands; then turn it over and once again take a deep breath. Bring your attention to the space you are in and come back to the present moment

A Soul Beyond One Lifetime

It seems to me that when we say "our animals choose us," this really is often the case. In such occurrences animals are linking into the energy we shared with them many lifetimes ago. This past-life connection has expanded my sense of the soul and deepened my personal connection with every single animal. My personal experience of being a nonbeliever, then a skeptic, to an "experiencer" and a firm believer has enabled me to perceive myself as a spirit in a human body and not just a physical body with a mind. Now I genuinely believe both animals and humans share a spirit or soul beyond just one lifetime, and I feel that this can manifest again and again, especially with the latest addition to our family, our feral cat named Tippy. I am convinced my childhood cat Timmy sent Tippy to find me.

When establishing such connections through the healing of animals or communicating with them, this idea becomes more of a palpable reality. Identifying with the soul of an animal, more so than with the personality, can play a powerful role in total connection.

Tess

When our wonderful cat Tess passed away during the writing of this book, we were totally distraught. I cannot put into words the void we felt after her passing. Tess was a very special cat, one in a million, and as I write this small tribute my eyes are filled with tears. She was just ten days from her seventeenth birthday and had come to us as a rescue, aged eight.

When we lost our cat Tansie, aged sixteen, in 2006 (another rescue cat who wasn't expected to make it past her eighth birthday), we were in despair. I am committed to the realization that not long after Tansie's passing from spirit she had pointed us in the direction of Tess.

Tess shared nearly nine years with us, was a total house cat, and was a unique feline in every way. She demanded five meals a day, had the strangest meow, loved any visiting dogs (extraordinary, as she was scared of the dog within her previous family), and was so intense and in tune with my crystals collection. The strangest thing about Tess was that she was a replica of Tansie in almost every personality trait. They even passed away with the same condition.

Since Tess passed just six weeks ago at the time of writing this chapter, I nearly didn't continue with this book; but just like Tansie gave us Tess, I wanted to give you, the reader, something too, so I continued to write.

As animal connectors, we often find it incredibly difficult when companions leave us behind for their journey to Rainbow Bridge.

The day after Tess passed away I had to heal my spirit. I felt fragmented and unable to concentrate on daily life, let alone the writing of this book. I needed to look inwards for healing, and through personal journeys and connection I began to feel whole once more, knowing that we will see each other again.

Such personal inward journeys help expand our consciousness and awareness of our animals in spirit. They also help us release any emotions associated with their passing and our part within it. Often, we feel guilty about releasing our animal from pain, even though we know it may be the right thing to do. These feelings can be hard to shake. We may even experience guilt for allowing our animal to linger in their final days, longer than we really should have done. We may experience sadness because we weren't able to say goodbye in the way we wanted, or we may even feel sorry that we could not be there in their final moments.

The exercise below will help ease your soul if you, like me, found the passing hard to come to terms with. This journey will help you to release and ground any feelings, worries, or concerns, too.

Step by Step—Rainbow Bridge Star Journey

Lie down in a safe and secure place, a place where you will not be disturbed.

Close your eyes and relax, and with every exhalation feel yourself becoming more and more at peace.

Now imagine that you are walking under the night sky. As you walk, you look up at the bright and radiant cosmos and notice the illuminating stars that light your way.

You become transfixed by their beauty and feel the need to lie down on the solid earth beneath the shining stars.

You begin to notice one star growing brighter and it beams directly upon you, surrounding you in its glowing, vibrant light. You experience a sense of freedom like never before and you feel uplifted in this radiant and majestic starlight.

Your heart begins to dance as you feel totally at one with the universal energy and your own guiding star.

As you lie upon the earth you feel your spirit lifted upwards by the force of this cosmic energy, and as you lie on the warm, dark ground a shooting star falls to the earth and lands about six inches above your heart.

Within the star a picture comes into view, almost like a photograph. As you gaze deeper into the star the image becomes clearer, and you see it's your beloved animal in spirit.

You feel your energy merging with the star, and the image within the star falls to meet the energy of your heart center.

You experience such a deep connection to your animal and you begin to speak to them, mind to mind, soul to soul. You speak of love, of sorrow, of gratitude, of guilt, of peace, of connection.

Allow your thoughts and feelings to be expressed to your wonderful animal from the starlight of Rainbow Bridge. Take as long as you need.

You know your thoughts have been heard and understood, and you begin to feel lighter in your heart, mind, and body.

You take a few deep, releasing breaths, and as you do so you become aware of a warm and golden glow surrounding your physical body.

From beneath your feet to the top of your head, you see a rainbow arc of light that is comforting and loving, and you know this comes from your animal in spirit.

The image of your animal on the star in front of you begins to absorb the rainbow arc of light and you begin to see it move upwards, back up into the cosmos; yet you do not feel sad, as you know you will meet with them again.

As you look upwards you see the brightest star in the whole of the sky: your animal.

Inhale with a deep, grounding breath and open your eyes whenever you feel ready to do so.

Tansie—Alias Psychic Moon

Personally, I held on to feelings of guilt in relation to my cat Tansie even when Tess entered our lives. Tansie was also known as "Psychic Moon," as she was the most spiritually aware cat that we have ever encountered. Just like Tess, Tansie was a larger lady feline, and at the time she came into my life I was working as a fundraiser and home inspector for Sheffield Hallam Cats Protection League. Through their charity leader I became aware of two tabby cats who were looking for a special indoor home: Tansie, aged seven, and her daughter Tabitha, aged five. They were being rehomed as their owner, David, had recently lost his wife and had four other cats to care for, as well as being registered disabled.

A few months prior to hearing about Tansie and Tabitha, my rescue cat Sophie (the remarkable shrew catcher!) died from leukemia, and I just didn't know if I could open my heart so soon to another cat. So I decided I would just go to "look" at Tansie and Tabitha, without making a commitment. However, when both cats began grooming each other and purring loudly upon my lap, I instantly fell in love with both of them. It was obvious that Tabitha was very vocal, as every time I posed a question to her, she had to answer me; this went on for ages! I am sure there was a little Siamese in her somewhere. David explained how the six cats were all related, and it was obvious that he loved them all very much and was finding it hard to part with Tansie and Tabitha.

David took out some photographs of the two cats when they were kittens. He then showed me the cat "family tree" he had on the wall. I was smitten, and although David found it hard to surrender these two girls, Tansie and Tabitha came home with me that very evening. I can't begin to describe how my life became enriched once more by these two tabby felines. Tansie was a brown tabby and a Taurean; a laid-back, placid cat, happiest when she had a full plate of food in front of her. Tabitha was a mackerel and white tabby, a Gemini, and a real chatterbox, happiest when she could have the last word!

After a few weeks, Tansie reinforced my childhood beliefs that all animals are psychic. I'd be engrossed in one task or another when Tansie would walk into the room and all of a sudden an obscure thought would enter my mind. Not just a regular, everyday thought but a warning, a prophecy, or a psychic flash of insight. These incidents were more than just a coincidence, as they occurred every couple of weeks, always when Tansie caught my eye. Whenever this happened Tansie looked at me, blinked, and jerked her head as if in a nod to say, "You understand me." What transpired after each thought transference never ceased to amaze me. Friends would call to inform me of them not feeling well, or would call to say they were getting married or divorced, or to speak of redundancy and death. It was hard for me not to say, "I already know, Tansie just told me"; but how could I? I just feigned surprise and offered support wherever it was needed. She even alerted me to the forthcoming death of her daughter, Tabitha, who passed away from a recurrence of mammary tumors one year after she had undergone an invasive operation to remove the initial growths.

There then came a prophecy from Tansie, which included a treasured family member of mine, and I found this hard to accept. The nights were drawing in; it was late September, and I set the sticks to light a fire in our open grate. Tansie came into the room and lay across the back of the sofa. I became aware of a sense of uneasiness enveloping the room, and looking over my shoulder at Tansie, I saw that her head was hung low. The energy was heavy in the room, and instantly I received a thought about my Nan. In the pit of my stomach I felt that bad news would soon come and I knew all was not well with Nan. I tried shrugging off this feeling of foreboding, but I couldn't. Tansie blinked, nodded, and then jumped down from the sofa to join me beside the fire; I knew she was offering me comfort by her presence as I stroked her head. The tone of the telephone shattered the silence, and as I picked up the receiver I heard tears. It was my mother informing me that Nan had passed away an hour earlier. Nan had suffered from pancreatic cancer in the months leading up to her death, and as I sat in disbelief at the news, I knew she had at last been set free from this debilitating illness. Tansie had connected with this news too.

Years passed by and Tansie became ill herself. Tansie was not only special in regards to her ability to communicate spiritual and psychic messages to me, but also one very lucky cat in relation to her own well-being. She was born with a heart defect along with an enlarged thyroid gland. The latter had led her to easily gain weight, as her thyroid was unable to regulate her metabolism effectively. Initially it was expected that Tansie wouldn't reach the age of eight, and that the birth of Tabitha may have placed an extra strain on her heart; however, she amazed us all by how she carried on to the age of fifteen, regularly enjoying healing.

One summer's day I took Tansie to the vet, as I noticed she wasn't eating. Numerous blood tests concluded that her thyroid function was very erratic, and her heart was beating irregularly; her body was in physical decline. Armed with three lots of medication I came home and tried to make the best of a thoroughly upsetting situation. Sitting with Tansie, I cried; I could not bear the thought of losing her.

I gave Tansie her daily medication, which at first seemed to help, though it wasn't long before the medication stopped working altogether. I was too emotionally involved and deeply connected to Tansie to offer her healing at these final stages, and for weeks I sat with her, trying to coax her to eat, almost pleading with her. Often when we are personally emotionally attached to an animal, we can't separate our feelings from our energy, so we often are unable to give effective healing treatments due to the anxieties and worries coming through. I knew Tansie was fading, but I did not want to let her go. I asked myself many questions: "How will I cope without her? How will my spirit survive? How will I go on without her in my life?" I knew through reading her energy that her physical life here on earth was over, and she was telling me so. She was pleading with me to let her go, but I just couldn't.

I suffered with a guilt-laden conscience after Tansie had passed over. Through my own selfishness I had allowed Tansie to linger on in life, long after her spirit had faded. I was holding her back on earth *for me,* nothing more. The guilt I carried around was with me for a number of years, but in the end I learned a huge lesson from it. I will never let an animal carry on with an existence just to support myself and my unfounded fears, so consequently we allowed Tess to pass with dignity when she chose to; the timing was perfect. Life does carry on without them because they remain deeply in our hearts, and I know in my soul that I will see them all again. Wait for me.

Ways to Honor Their Memory

Unfortunately, when we lose a beloved companion, the only way to get to the other side of the pain and grief is to let yourself feel it and move through it. Time alone won't get you through the pain, overeating can't stop the pain, keeping busy won't make it go away, and watching TV won't erase your loss either. The only way to move through the process and to bring your grief to completion in a healthy way is to discover and communicate any unexpressed emotions you feel about your relationship with your pet. There is no set time frame for you to go through the grieving process. The length of time is different for every person. Even when you have recovered, that doesn't mean you won't ever miss your pet or that you won't still feel sad once in a while.

There are many things you can do to honor the memory of your pet and keep their vibration alive:

- Plant a tree or shrub in their favorite place.
- Make a scrapbook or photo album with pictures of you and your pet.
- Write a book about your pet, make a video, write a song or a poem, or draw a picture.

- Write about you and your pet in a journal to help you process your feelings.

- Erect a memory plaque in your garden.

- Make a donation to an animal rescue center in honor of your pet.

- Create a "memory box" containing photographs and some of the pet's favorite toys or other belongings, such as a collar, lead, food bowl, etc.

Spirit Never Dies

Personally, I have discovered that animals who pass away, whether due to natural causes or because they have been euthanized, have their souls go into a resting state for a period of time. This period seems to help them make the transition from their physical body into their pure spirit form. Many times an animal cannot be reached when you try to connect with them, so it's best to allow a little time before trying to make a connection. I constantly hear about those animals who have passed on continuing to watch over their household, and their families still feeling their essence around them.

My own animal bond has deepened greatly over the years and I have come to realize that it isn't just in this lifetime that we connect so deeply with them. We often bring the energy forwards from previous lives, becoming reunited once again, soul to soul.

My Dream Boy

As I approached the livery yard my stomach flipped. I'd been working as a professional animal therapist for over ten years, so I couldn't really understand why I felt so uneasy. When Mrs. Williams had booked me to give healing to her horse three weeks prior to my visit, I knew somehow that it wasn't going to be a straightforward session. I try not to have any preconceived ideas about any forthcoming treatment, but I just knew this particular session was going to be different.

I stepped out of the car and was met by a woman aged about sixty. What was most odd was the fact that she remarked "There's someone I would like you to meet." I started to become nervous, almost like a teenager on a first date, and as I approached the stable block I stopped to take a few deep breaths, which was most unlike me. I walked past six or seven horses and slowly approached the last stable. For some reason I stopped short, not daring look inside. Instead I stood rigid and proceeded to take out a consultation form from my case. As Mrs. Williams was giving me of all the relevant health details in relation to this horse in the stable, the energy that consumed me became a little disjointed, and I started to become edgy. As I tried to gather my thoughts, and as I put pen to paper, I felt an overwhelming warmth and so much love wash over me; a deep peacefulness and connection like I'd never felt before. You could say I felt like I had "come home."

When I placed my pen back in my folder and looked up from the consultation form, I saw the most amazing horse looking back at me from over the stable door. "Here's your boy. This is Dream," said Mrs. Williams. Another rather odd thing to say, I thought, but somehow I knew exactly what she meant. Dream's eyes widened and they never left my gaze; we became instantly connected and his energy felt oddly familiar.

I had been asked to give Dream healing on an emotional level, as Mrs. Williams felt that there had always been a "missing link" somewhere in his life, like something causing emotional upset, almost as if he was searching for something he had lost in the past. As I dowsed with my small brass pendulum over the selection of crystals I had taken with me, Mrs. Williams told me how she had stumbled across my website quite by accident. She said how as soon as she saw my photograph, Dream had popped into her head and he'd nodded in approval about her contacting me. This gave her the prompt to call me that very evening, knowing that Dream's missing link mystery was going to be solved.

With the help of my pendulum I selected my crystals: chrysanthemum stone, jade, and selenite. I showed each one in turn to Dream and he gave me a knowing look along with an approving head nod. I cleansed my hands, grounded myself, and connected to Dream at soul level by placing both of my hands upon his butterfly chakra. I then placed each crystal in turn directly onto his body, channeling their energy. Dream's spirit was pulling my hands deeper within his body and I felt like my mind was turning the pages of a book, there was so much information. His butterfly chakra was vibrating greatly with the energy of jade as I pressed this closely to his heart. My third eye, in the center of my forehead, along with my crown chakra, started to pulsate and whirl and I felt the reality of time become suspended. I circled the chrysanthemum stone around Dream's butterfly chakra and could feel the energy rhythmically expanding into the whole of his auric field; we were both pulsating. I instinctively knew there was a blockage of energy being cleared around his heart chakra, as the crystal in my palm began to draw it outwards.

Past-Life Visions

I couldn't possibly have prepared myself for what happened next. I left my physical body in the stable and I saw myself sitting upon a majestic dappled horse, riding through a dense and dark leafy forest. The rain fell heavily and hard and I could smell the aroma of both fern and oak. The dappled horse was heavily laden with my belongings and as we rode onwards, the air surrounding us felt tense. Within my vision something had come loose from the horse's panniers. My eyes fell to the ground and I turned this stunning stallion around to retrieve the lost item. It was then that my majestic companion fell to the ground and let out a shattering cry that pierced the forest. My beautiful steed had been shot with six arrows, yet I could see no person.

The chrysanthemum stone I held dropped from my hand and brought me back to the present moment in time. Dream's muscles became taut and rigid, and as I gathered my thoughts I picked up a piece of selenite to help discharge any residual energy surrounding him. He let out an almighty sigh and began to violently move his head up and down, and I knew that somehow I needed to maintain physical contact during this strange episode. As I rested my hand on his withers an obscure word came to my mind, quickly followed by another vision: I saw myself sitting on the woodland floor, sobbing at the sight of my dying horse and repeating the word "ashleeng."

Dream started to neigh, which snapped me back into my physical body. A shiver coursed through this equine client and Mrs. Williams began to sob. I disconnected from healing and grounded the energy that surrounded this magnificent horse. Dream suddenly looked at me and his owner with an "all knowing" look.

Mrs. Williams knew that a great shift in her horse's emotional energy had taken place. She said she could physically see the release of stagnant, emotional energy leaving his body. My work with Dream was over.

Returning home I needed to know more, and began to research the word "ashleeng." I was astounded at my discovery. "Ashleeng" has a strong association with "Aisling," a Celtic word and name meaning "dream"! This profound discovery began to make so much sense. After many inward journeys and dreams, it was confirmed that Dream was my old horse from a past life.

It happened like this. One year prior to this session with Dream, I had undergone a past-life regression. The regression uncovered a previous lifetime in medieval Wales; the year was 1256. During the regression, I spoke about riding a dappled gray horse through dense, woodland undergrowth when tragedy stuck. So I knew my previous lifetime involved Dream, and I know that part of his soul had remained attached to me for over eight hundred years. Furthermore, Mrs. Williams recognized that Dream connected with this too.

Shortly after my visit with Dream I was notified that Mrs. Williams had passed away. Her husband explained that he felt it had been her mission to find the right healing for Dream before she passed over, and she even left a legacy to a national equine charity honoring her special horse, Dream.

Past Lives, Current Love

Initially, back when I studied psychology, I was dismissive of the whole concept of past lives. To me it seemed a fanciful idea, one that did not have any scientific evidence as its base. However, I have come to understand that not everything can be scientifically proven.

The concept of past lives makes perfect sense because of the cyclical form of every aspect of nature: life, death, and rebirth. When a tree loses its foliage in winter, it retreats within until the spring, to be born again, regrowing buds and foliage, only to die again in autumn. In most nature-based faiths, the whole concept of past lives becomes a vital part of understanding how we can connect with ourselves and with animals who have passed over.

Many years ago I trained as a past-life regression therapist, and since then I have experienced far too many regressions that can't be passed off as merely coincidental or put down to creative imaginations. I wholeheartedly believe in the past lives of humans and animals.

Until we meet again…

In Conclusion

If there's one thing I've learned from animals, it's that we never stop learning! The animal kingdom has so much to offer and to teach; so much more than we could ever begin to understand. Throughout my career, I've been richly blessed to meet many human beings that instinctively know how holistic techniques can dramatically enhance the lives of their animals and bring about enrichment and joy. I hope you, dear reader, can enjoy putting into practice the various techniques I've presented within this book. In healing, we work with unconditional love, and this is all we seek—human and animal. Thank you for sharing this remarkable and memorable journey with me.

To Write the Author

If you wish to contact the author or would like more information about this book, please write to the author in care of Llewellyn Worldwide, and we will forward your request. Both the author and publisher appreciate hearing from you and learning of your enjoyment of this book and how it has helped you. Llewellyn Worldwide cannot guarantee that every letter written to the author can be answered, but all will be forwarded. Please write to:

Niki J. Senior
℅ Llewellyn Worldwide
2143 Wooddale Drive
Woodbury, MN 55125-2989

Please enclose a self-addressed stamped envelope for reply,
or $1.00 to cover costs. If outside the USA, enclose
an international postal reply coupon.

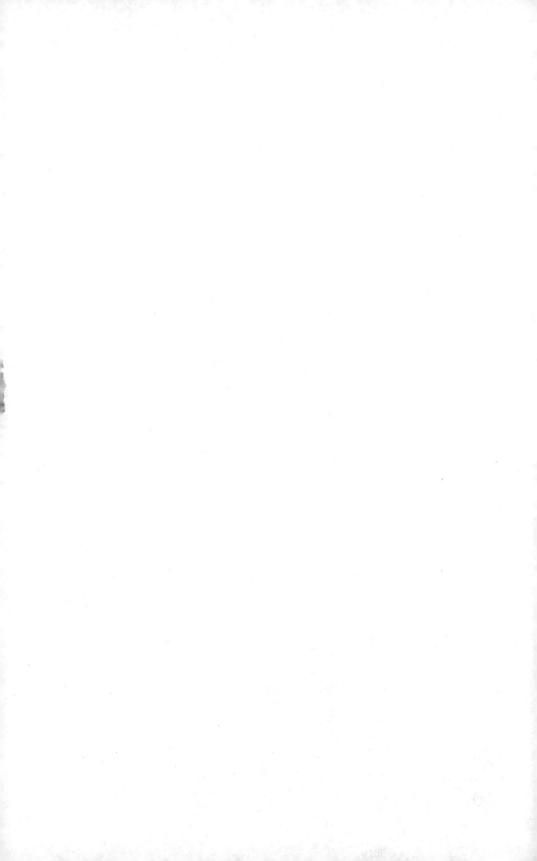